WAITING TO DIE, RUNNING TO LIVE

Michael Patrick Burke

I.H.S. Publishers

Saint Louis, Missouri

TABLE OF CONTENTS

WAITING TO DIE, RUNNING TO LIVE

"In covering sports and athletes for many years, I've observed many amazing athletic performances, but Mike Burke's accomplishments as a marathon runner with a debilitating chronic illness stand out as a most amazing feat from which we can all take away valuable life lessons."

~Zip Rzeppa,
TV Sportscaster and Author

"If you are trying to live a more positive life—then this book is a must read. Mike shows how Positive Intelligence really works, and when applied in daily activities, it can really make a huge impact."

~Matt Cowell, MBA
President, Ascend Business Strategies

I.H.S. Publishers
3920 S. Old Hwy. 94, Suite 36
St. Charles, MO 63304
(636) 447-6000

Editor: Kelly Boutross
Front Cover Design: Mike Donovan
Compositor: Trese Gloriod

Printed in the United States of America

ISBN: 978-0-9847656-3-8

INTRODUCTION

Once I had a dear friend in college, Melissa, earn an A on a paper. The assignment was to be a short autobiography. Being a chronic procrastinator, my friend did not prepare her paper in advance. Just before class started, on the due date for the assignment, she wrote these—and only these—autobiographical words: *I am succinct.* For cleverness and creativity, she received the highest grade. For last-minute shenanigans, she received a stern warning from her professor.

I, on the other hand, am not succinct—but I do have the attention span of a Schnauzer. Not much can hold my attention for more than 10 minutes. As a result, this book is broken up into a series of stories, each based on key moments in my life. They are in chronological order so you can follow events easily. Take each period in my life one at a time or as a whole. See if my stories can help you make a positive and even life-changing influence on yourself, your family, co-workers, friends, and those you will never meet. My life has been full of moments that have been difficult to prepare for. I have used these moments to better understand myself and others in my life.

Why is my life worth reading about? Perhaps because by reasonable medical expectations I should be dead, and by societal standards I should be a broken man. I am neither dead nor broken. In fact, I'm thriving and embracing life. Everyone will experience the things I've experienced and come to know in some degree. Some will get a little dose, while others will get an overdose. My story isn't about being in the grips of despair and hopelessness and then breaking free. It's about how I, with much support from family, friends, co-workers, and strangers alike, avoided the deepest pitfalls of despair.

What This Book Is *Not* About

This book is not about running and triathlons any more than it is about living with my particular set of circumstances. My experiences can be applied to whatever area of your life you see fit, and will help you to embrace whatever challenges you face. This book is also not about me living perfectly or having all the answers. I am just a regular guy. I think it is important to know that we don't have to BE somebody special in the eyes of the world to DO something extraordinary. What I *do* know is this: I have lived day-to-day and year-to-year staring down very limited expectations for my life, and I've managed to do that remaining even more positive and determined to thrive than I could dare to hope as a young man.

In the spirit of my good friend the clever procrastinator—and my canine attention span—let's get on with my stories.

Chapter 1

WHY SHARE DEEPLY PERSONAL STORIES?

"A man that flies from his fear may find that he has only taken a shortcut to meet it."

J.R.R. Tolkien, novelist

I am writing this book because life with a chronic illness can be lonely. Even surrounded by a loving family and support-ive friends, there is a feeling of isolation. When you live with a life-threatening condition, you don't want to be a burden... to *anyone*. You especially don't want to burden the people closest to you. You assume they have enough on their plates, so you don't let the very people who love you most in on your thoughts. Not only do you not want to be a burden, but you have the added desire of wanting to be a strong example for them. Sharing your fearful or sad thoughts is the last thing you want to do. You must always be strong, even when you're not feeling confident or strong. Whether it's internal thoughts or worrying about money or insurance or bills, you don't want to make others worry... so you don't.

As suffering people, we end up putting ourselves on an island. Interiorly, we scream at the top of our lungs: "You don't understand me!" "You can't *possibly* know what it's like to be me!" We believe this so strongly that we don't just create an island, but an island fortress. This fortress is impenetrable to the good advice, love, and encouragement of others. These wonderful things bounce off us like a rubber ball hitting a stone wall. To make matters worse, we even begin to be proud that we are alone. While internal strength is a must, the fortresses we build repel people, their kindness, and their insights.

I also write because living with a chronic condition is an everyday, non-stop, around-the-clock experience. There is no break from the effects it has on your body, and it can be exasperating. There is not a single minute in any day when you are not reminded of your condition. Whether you experience pain from the condition, or you take medicine throughout every day, there is no mental break—and it can wear on you. Your condition ends up consuming your entire life. It often seems like there is no light at the end of the tunnel, and if you let your guard down for even a short time, the consequences may be fatal.

Here's the ultimate reason for this book: there *is* a way out of the isolation, fear, negativity, and the daily grind that living with great challenges presents. I write because there is a life-changing result that comes when you take life's challenges head on, and I want to share how I experienced this. I stopped making life decisions based on the expectation that my life would be shortened. Before I developed this mindset, I essentially allowed myself to think the best things in life wouldn't happen to me; I was only waiting for something bad to happen. This book is really the story of how I did a "mental 180-degree turn."

I've experienced this conquering feeling and resulting change many times in my life, and it comes in both "victories" and "defeats," sometimes even several in a single day. The image of a finish line always provides the end to any new goal, and also provides a feeling of great accomplishment. The daily journey to the finish line is just as important. Every day that I do something to take care of my body and mind, I get the reward of making a difference in my own life, along with a little extra peace of mind. Running *away* from my life (in my younger years) and running *toward* my life (in my later years) will be a constant theme in the stories in this book. My first "run" created

4

regret and unrest, and the other "run" gave me a deeper sense of who I am and what I needed to do.

To explain the feeling of personal victory over one's challenges, I would like to introduce you to a famous photo I've come across. This image illustrates how I feel about living beyond expectations with a deadly disease. In this photo, Mohammed Ali stands over Sonny Liston. Sonny Liston is on the floor of the boxing ring, flat on his back. His arms are resting on the floor, stretched above his head. His head is turned toward Ali, and it would appear he is calmly watching "The Champ." (Or perhaps he wasn't looking at Ali at all, but staring off into the stars, as he was just knocked out!) Ali is standing at Liston's feet. He is towering over Liston with his mouth wide open, yelling. As the stage lights shine on his massive figure, Ali has his arm cocked across his torso in a manner that lets the viewer see the strength of the force which has knocked Liston to the floor. "The Greatest" is reveling in his victory and in this fight has supreme mastery over Liston.

When I picture myself in this famous snapshot, I'm not standing over a human opponent, but over this disease. I dominated! I punched, kicked, scratched, and had a knock-down, drag-out street brawl with a deadly disease—and I beat it. No "Marquess of Queensberry" rules applied to this grudge match. (By the way, the Marquess of Queensberry rules have governed boxing matches since 1865 and ensure a "gentlemanly" match. Well, when it comes to my fight with this disease, I ain't no gentleman—so the Marquess Of Queensberry has been nowhere to be seen in my life!)

My goal? To stand over life with supreme confidence, knowing I've lived well. There's no doubt I won. In this match of life, I've been knocked down; I've been worn out, bruised, sweaty, and weary. But I've never been beaten. I've pushed hard in my life to do more because of my challenges. I understand that by not just accepting the challenges I face, but embracing them, I am made stronger. The very things that frustrate, anger, and upset me also provide constant reassurance that I have a unique purpose in this world. Since I can't change genetics, all I can change is the way I fight. The battle is mental, physical, and spiritual... and by God, my intent is to come out on the fulfilled side of this life!

Embracing my fears, pain, and challenges brings focus, creativity, and purpose to life's daily grind. During training for a race that I will discuss later, I printed shirts that said "Embrace the Pain." For me, this phrase had dual meaning. I would be "suffering" for 18 weeks of training, building my strength to be able to complete 70.3 miles of continuous motion. That slogan also meant that by not only *accepting* my life with a chronic medical condition, but also *embracing* this life, I could concentrate on living life to its fullest. A year later I was reading an article by two-time world Ironman Champion Chris McCormack, and he talked about this very topic. I was astonished that he used nearly the same three words I did. He called it "embracing the suck." I almost fell out of my chair wondering how a world-class athlete and a middle-of-the-pack, amateur competitor could come to the same conclusion about winning. Whether we're talking about a sporting competition or living life with no regrets, the same thought process applies. I was greatly inspired to discover that this is a universal truth, and I want *you* to experience the exasperating yet wonderful battle of "embracing the challenge."

Finally, I write this book because of the following Facebook post. It comes from one of the strongest-willed people I have had contact with. As you will read later, the disease that wreaks havoc on my body has also devastated hers, but it has also developed a very strong spirit within her. Here is her post:

"UPDATE: I got home yesterday. I am sooo weak. I tried to walk up just two steps from my garage to the house and collapsed. Then I stood up and tried again and fell. I'm pale, thin, and very depressed. I'm finding it very hard to see the light at the end of the tunnel. I keep thinking about transplant and what a daunting road it is. I wonder if I have it in me… if it's worth the struggle for my loved ones as well as doubting my own stamina. I don't want to bankrupt my family trying to save me. My mom needs shoulder surgery now. She can't be 4 different people. I keep thinking about people like _____ and _____ that fought back from weak places to get their lung transplant. HOW did you do it? Where did you start when you can barely walk to begin with?"

She got through that difficult period with flying colors. Two things were vivid to me as this was unfolding. First, aside from the difficult day she posted this on Facebook, she has maintained a great deal of internal strength and has been an inspiration to others for years. Second, this cross would have been so much harder for her if she had not received a great deal of support from her friends. In her time of need, I saw her people come to her side with a multitude of positive thoughts, prayers, and offers of help. She is so fortunate to have people remind her how important she is to them. I wonder if she knows that it is her struggle that uplifts those around her. Let me correct that—it is her *approach* to her struggle that uplifts those around her, and in turn provides her with support.

For those without a chronic illness but are witness to someone with challenges, I want you to know you can get in the fight with those around you, and as a result experience your life to the fullest. I want you to experience what it is like to deeply impact another person and have your life changed because you did something uncomfortable and difficult. Our day of reckoning is coming, and it is nothing to be frightened of if you did all that is within you to live well... and then just a little more. We will be fulfilled when we know we have embraced all aspects of our life, eased the fight for the people around us, and made a difference.

As A Last Thought...

Another reason I have written these stories for others to read is because each time I have shared them, I have been rewarded in some way. I told you I was like a Schnauzer, and just like a canine, I will work for treats. Those treats come from kids in underprivileged areas, who through my story see that greater things are possible even though a tough road is ahead. The rewards come from a teenager who took comfort from knowing I had the same thoughts she had at 16, but I have come out on the good side of things and lived "to tell the tale." The reward also comes from listening to people suffering from a different physical or mental affliction who just need a little encouragement. All these people can relate to my story. The rewards come from connecting to those wanting to discover a greater purpose for themselves. I have found myself in a unique position to listen and offer encouragement. The best part of all this, and the piece you must always keep at your core, is that the outcome begins and ends with *you*. Isn't that awesome? YOU have the final say about how to live and what to think. And no one can take that privilege and right away from you.

Now you know why I feel compelled to share such deep and personal experiences, when a mere few years ago, I wouldn't even talk about my condition to the people I should have trusted the most.

Are you ready for some stories? I have a million tales (like any good Irishman), but my attention span wouldn't stand for *too* much explanation. I'll do my best, though, in the pages of this book.

Chapter 2

THE GUN BARREL

*"I am not the product of my circumstances.
I am a product of my decisions."*

Stephen Covey, author and motivational speaker

I'm 44 years old. I own a small business. I'm married. I own a house. I run marathons and triathlons for health benefits. If you think that sounds like a fairly typical life, you'd be right. I do live a typical life, except for the fact that I was expected to die some 30 years ago—and that was being optimistic. After being diagnosed with a fatal genetic disease, I was expected to live no longer than five years. In 1971, the disease I was diagnosed with didn't have more than a handful of survivors beyond kindergarten. At first glance, my life is very typical. Throw in a fatal chronic disease that there is no cure for, and the ballgame changes.

Since my diagnosis at 14 months old, children suffering from this disease have started living just a little bit longer. The obvious result of this is a longer life expectancy. At the age of 14 months, I was diagnosed and given a maximum of five years to live. By the time I turned five years old, my life expectancy was adjusted to seven years old. By the time I turned seven, my life expectancy was nine. When I was nine, my life expectancy was 11. When I was 17, the life expectancy turned to 19. On my 23rd birthday, the life expectancy was 25... and so on until my 30th birthday. I'm sure you can understand how difficult it must have been with all those "years" and "expectancies" constantly hanging over my head.

When you are 16 years old and come to the realization that your body has an expiration date of 18 years, you get quite a jolt. At 16 I became fully aware of my precarious situation, and for the next 15 years I felt I was staring down the barrel of a loaded gun. Think of an action movie in which the hero suddenly notices a tiny red dot squarely placed on his chest. This red dot is from a laser scope, which happens to be attached to a high-powered rifle. As the audience, we feel two things in that split second. Our first emotion is a strong sense of impending doom, felt on behalf of our hero. The second emotion is the need to react quickly. There is an immediate sense to *get moving*... or else. Our hero doesn't have time to plan out his move. The hero simply reacts, and whatever happens is always better than getting "whacked." That mix of impending doom and my compelling desire to do something immediately became very urgent when I fully realized the extent of my health situation. The likelihood of early death was unavoidable and you were constantly reminded of that fact, especially if you were involved with fund-raising or had constant contact with the small community of people also suffering from the disease.

The toughest aspect of my whole situation was the figure of my life expectancy; it was always moving and just in front of me. In some ways, however, living like I did is like the proverbial horse and carrot. The carrot dangles in front of the horse, motivating the horse to constantly plod on. Instead of a carrot, I was looking at death. Death is a hell of a thing to be dangling in front of you. The prospect of dying as a primary motivator creates much negativity. In addition, having death always looming in front of you blocks your vision. It is very difficult to see through the immediate prospect of dying; it is a struggle to see a future full of possibilities and a life that has purpose.

It is natural to think the incremental increases in life expectancy were something positive in an otherwise desperate situation. If you're thinking from a parental or caretaker standpoint, you are right. My parents and doctors took great encouragement from this fact. While it was perhaps something to hold onto, the fact remained that the clinical outlook was undeniably death at a young age. For me, to say the least, it was frustrating. My disease often looked insurmountable.

From all of this life-expectancy talk, hospital stays, and vast amounts of medicine I took grew a level of fear that would in-fluence my decisions for a great many years. I didn't possess an overwhelming fear. Fear did not drive me to drugs, destructive behavior, or pervasive thoughts that life itself was not worth living. While in high school, my fear manifested itself as *apathy*. I didn't see why I should make an effort to excel, as the time line for me was very short. Apathy eventually evolved into urgency, and from college-age on I felt compelled to do "stuff" before it was too late. That urgency would result in some of the best and worst moments in my life. Upon embracing my life with this disease, this urgency turned to a *drive* that came from a place of purpose instead of a place of fear. Working with a purpose is when I started living a fulfilling life.

I believe that, if allowed to, this fear could have completely overtaken my thoughts and led to the worst behavior one can imagine. I firmly believe that I have been blessed time and again with a strong, positive attitude and fervor to overcome obstacles in life. That will to overcome difficulties is a gift from God, and it has been aided by a lifetime of positive influential people and my own decision to wrap my arms around this life and see it as a blessing versus a curse. Throughout this book you will be introduced to some of the greatest people I've known. Through their fellowship, I have learned what I now know. Without their influence, I don't know if I would have discovered how to live happily.

What is it that I learned to do? Read on...

Embrace the Challenge

My greatest desire for this book is that it will help you to get a glimpse of what it is like to overcome challenges. My hope is that you can learn to embrace the challenges in your own life. Whether it is a life-threatening illness or just a difficult situation at work or home, by embracing the obstacles in your life, you will begin to find positive solutions and new opportunities.

Perspective

Putting our challenges into proper perspective will help you to enjoy life more. Just when I'm getting most frustrated at my physical condition, I inevitably come across somebody who is suffering on an even greater level, and my attitude is corrected quickly. It's not that I feel better because they are worse off than I am. Rather, observing others simply provides a perspective of gratitude for the great things I *do* have, and these folks inspire me to embrace life despite its challenges; maybe even *because* of its challenges.

Purpose

Know that your life has *purpose*, and live knowing that your actions have purpose. The realization of having true purpose will be sustaining during those times when sheer will is all that gets us through.

Do It For Others

If it were not for a steady stream of positive people in my life, I don't know if I would be alive. If I did manage to live, I'm certain I would not have accomplished the wonderful things I have. I certainly wouldn't be in the "1% Club." (One percent being the percentage of the United States population who will complete a full marathon race.)

"Clinical" Isn't Me

Clinically speaking, I don't know anything about psychology—and I'm not pretending to know. You won't find clinical advice in this book in any way. What I do have to share is 44 years of life experience. When I talk to others living with some challenge, we somehow connect. While I can't give you clinical advice, you will come to realize what others are thinking and feeling. You will also learn what I did to face my challenges. You will also see what others did to help me. What you do with that knowledge makes all the difference. If you feel professional guidance will build on what I can tell you, I encourage you to seek that additional perspective.

Is This For Everyone?

I sincerely hope so. In this book, I'm not going to tell you right away the name of the medical condition that has influenced my life. I hear time and again from people of all ages that "nobody gets me…" and I've said these same words many times in the past. I assumed my particular set of circumstances created a block to all other humans' understanding of me. You might already be thinking: I don't have that kind of challenge, so why should I read this book? What you're going to read will make sense even when approaching ordinary challenges in work and family life. I encourage you to stay with me while I tell a story that is about a life less common in its particular details, but universal in its struggles.

We have a unique capacity and desire to *relate* to one another. The human heart is designed primarily for *relationships*. Why else would movies, books, plays, TV shows, and music fill us with emotions about what happened to people we have never met? Let's face it: most entertainment is about fictional characters, yet we still feel deep emotions about their plight. Who doesn't cry when Old Yeller's master is forced to kill his beloved dog? We cry over the death of a fictional dog. This "phenomenon" is either really bizarre or something very special.

Going Deep

We are also wired for compassion. I'm talking about something greater than tolerance, sympathy, or even empathy. These ideas are good things, but we are born with a sense of compassion for one another, and that is what we must deepen. Compassion, by definition, encompasses sympathy and empathy and takes it to a whole new level. Naturally, then, compassion is a more difficult objective, but when we take on the responsibility and courage of compassion we change people and ourselves.

Even the most successful and happy people I know have had challenges to overcome. Our own challenges can be simple or complex. One way or another, we will all face some hurdle in life. My personal experience regarding challenge has been to either avoid it or face it head on. Whether your obstacle is mental, spiritual, emotional, or physical, I encourage you to embrace whatever comes your way. What great and inspiring story ends with someone running way?

The Long Haul

Life is short, but paradoxically, it is also a "long haul." I've had to take a ridiculous amount of medication from the day I was diagnosed with a fatal disease as an infant. I will have to take a ridiculous amount of medicine until I die or until this disease is cured. The good things we do for ourselves and others must be done over a *lifetime*. Staying focused at work for a lifetime is hard. Keeping your husband or wife feeling loved for a lifetime is truly difficult. Raising children is super difficult. Working out, eating right, and staying healthy is also a true challenge. Keeping a strong faith can be work, work, work.

But before we get going with the rest of my story, let me ask: is career success, raising awesome children, staying happily married, and walking with God worth work, and even a little pain? If you don't think so, I urge you to read on. If, on the other hand, you know that to be true, keep reading and you will enjoy a reminder of the awesome gifts we have.

The Importance of Humor

Where would I be without tons of fun in my life? They say that laughter is the best medicine, and there is much truth to that saying. Life has to be filled with funny and embarrassing moments as well as a host of characters that make life light-hearted. I've been blessed with all these things, and sometimes more embarrassing moments than I'd like to admit.

Aside from the "medicine" of humor, there are also a great many things I can do to make life easier from a physical standpoint. It seems to me that the older I get, the more therapies and medicines there are to take. Is this good or bad? Much like the rest of my life with a chronic disease, there are *two* sides to the medicine story.

Chapter 3

COMPLIANT

"Resistance is futile."

The Borg [Star Trek]

I'm a pretty positive-thinking fellow. I don't complain much about life with this disease, but this next bit is a sore spot. Please pardon my inability to control my emotions on this topic. Witnessing my temper tantrums actually might be amusing for you.

Let me get to my first rant: just hearing the word "compliant" makes me want to scream. The very definition of compliant makes most people squirm. Check it out:

Com • pli • ant: *conforming to requirements*

Synonyms: *obedient, submissive, docile*

When you were a teenager, would you be excited to be described as compliant? Docile? I didn't think so. My friends with children tell me this disgust for compliance begins very early. So just imagine having to be "compliant" as an adult.

I wish I could say I've overcome my natural resistance to taking all the medicine that is prescribed for my condition. It is still a battle to remain 100% in the right frame of mind to stay "compliant." At least now I see the point to taking it all. As a kid, I just thought it was pointless because my life expectancy was so short. Being "compliant" means taking *all* your medicine and doing *all* your therapies *all* the time. Check out what my day consists of in terms of compliance. (Imagine developing a habit to never forget all these meds and actually working in the time.) Also, imagine realizing as a kid that this is what you will have to do for the rest of your life... every *single* day:

(8) Zenpep™ per meal (To digest food—so you don't starve to death.)

(4) Zenpep™ with snacks

(1) Pantoprazole™ (Anti-acid, to balance the acid in your stomach so you don't get ulcers.)

(2) Vitamin D (Even though you take Zenpep™ your body still only extracts a fraction of the nutritional value from food.)

(1) Multivitamin (Again, you need pure nutrients because the body is so inefficient with processing food.)

(1) Lisinopril™ (To protect the liver... because diabetes is another "bonus" of the disease.)

(1) Insulin pump (Like I mentioned above, the pancreas fails and you may become insulin-dependent.)

That's thirty-six pills a day, not to mention having to wear a medical device. These aren't small pills like aspirin. Enzymes are huge pills that kids have to take as soon as possible. We still haven't touched on maintaining the lungs, neglect of which poses the greater threat to life. My lungs don't require so many pills, but they do require much more time.

(5) minutes – (1) time per day: Pulmozyme™ (This is an aerosol or "breathed-in" treatment to thin mucus in the lungs.)

(30) minutes – (2) times per day: Vibrating Vest (This vest is attached to an air compressor and shakes your upper body to break loose the mucus.)

(10) minutes – (2) times per day: TOBI™ (This is another aerosol treatment which is an antibiotic to kill the germs trapped by thick mucus.)

(5) minutes – (2) times per day: HyperSal™ (This is another aerosol treatment that makes the mucus more "moveable" through the airways, so you can spit it out if needed.)

When I review this list, the image I get is juggling. Juggling six flaming tennis balls, while riding a unicycle, while being chased by tigers, while calculating the theory of relativity and

reciting the alphabet backwards. Maybe not *that* complicated...
but sometimes it feels that way.

Grand Summary

Pills Per Day: 36   Pills Per Year: 13,140
Time Per Day Attached to Machine: 90 minutes
Time Per Year Attached to Machine: 32,850 minutes
or 547.5 hours

The Cost of Compliance...

You might be thinking... so what, it's only 90 minutes a
day. Just wake up a little early or do it before bed. You are absolutely correct. To that I'd say, YOU do this every day for the
rest of YOUR life. Only if you experience it yourself will you be
able to fully empathize with the great inconvenience a routine
like this creates. If you miss a day of this medical routine, you
will cough and get a sore belly. If you miss a few days, you will
develop a persistent cough and diarrhea. If you miss any significant number of days, you run the risk of catching a germ that
could land you in the hospital, or worse, kill you. If you miss a
significant amount of days of digestive enzymes you will start
losing weight. You may be thinking: big deal—I am *trying* to
lose weight anyway! People try to lose weight all over the world.
Well get this... there is a direct correlation between weight loss
and lung function loss, so losing weight is not an option; besides,
without the medication you would live with around-the-clock
diarrhea, which I can assure you is not a pleasant experience.

Now think how difficult it can be to fit 90 minutes of down-
time into your day. Most people struggle to find an additional
30 minutes to do a daily task. Now try to do it while going to
college full time or working a career and raising a family. Try
adding 30 minutes of exercise to everything we just outlined,
because exercise is the best therapy you can possibly do. I think
you get the picture of how frustrating it becomes when anybody
asks why you're not being compliant. I know those that ask if
I am taking my medicine are only thinking of my health—but
good Lord, it sure isn't easy to get all that done.

Sometimes you just want a break from it.

Mothers and Compliance

I know it's perhaps the most unfair thing in the world, but

here is the ugly truth: Mom, you can never ask me if I'm taking my medicine or going to the doctor. My wife can ask. My dad can ask. My brothers can ask. My friends can ask and my doctor can ask. Mom, you cannot! It's completely and utterly irrational, but that is how it is. It's almost cruel because Mom should be the one person that has the right to ask. For me, Mom should be the person that I appreciate the most *for* asking. My mother was the one that went to every doctor visit for 18 years. She worried the most. She loved me unconditionally when I was a teenager and manipulated her feelings. She loved me unquestioningly when I moved 1,000 miles from home for no reason other than I wanted to live a little before I died. If it came to a bitter end, she would be there for me after everyone else couldn't or wouldn't.

From the deepest part of my soul I ask forgiveness from all the mothers who can't ask "the question." I also want you to know that it is *not* personal. Your child loves you and when they get older and realize what you have meant in their life, they will finally be grateful. Keep loving and supporting your children— it is the most honorable duty on earth, even if it sometimes feels like it is also the most thankless!

Doctors and Compliance

Pssst. Hey, Doc. I have a secret to tell you. I hate coming to see you! You always tell me bad news. You always tell me I have to be doing more. Simply by visiting your office, I am reminded that I live with something so life-threatening I have to see you four times a year, even if I seem perfectly healthy. When I come to see you, I'm reminded that my body is on a precarious edge; we are looking for things that kill. You send me to get x-rays and blood work. You make me spit "loogies" into a cup and breathe into machines. You send in a social worker to make sure I'm "coping." It's very difficult to visit your office.

What's worse is that when I leave, I have nothing but time to think about what just went down. On the drive home I'm getting myself psyched up. I'm fighting the urge to be mad and upset at my circumstances. I don't want to obsess about decreased lung function or losing weight or the nasty germs spreading in my body. I surely don't want to bring the bad news home to my wife. I hate seeing the look of dread on her face, even though she is so supportive and strong. God help us if she were actually in the exam room listening to all the stuff going on with my body. I've had a lifetime to harden my emotions and brace for the "routine" clinic visit. She has not.

Hey Doc, I don't hate *you*. You've spent great effort, money, and time to be the best at diagnosing what's wrong with my body. I am thankful for you. I could never be an M.D. But you always tell me I have to be doing better. You tell me how insidious this disease is and that if I don't stay "compliant," the worst will happen. I know you are just doing your job when you tell me these things, but it doesn't make it any easier to hear. I cannot be treated like a machine that you just take in information about and process without an emotional response. I want to be treated as a human being exactly like yourself.

My Special Challenges with Doctors-in-Training

I once had a student doctor come into my exam room; without pause, he started in with the bad news. How I wasn't doing everything possible and how it would end up killing me. He went on and on, and when I wasn't responding in the manner he wished, this young man reminded me how he didn't care if I was being "compliant." He was just here to tell me how it was and the consequences of not following the rules. The words in my head were like this: "Guess what, I don't give a %$#@ about you either—so we're even." "I think I know what the consequences are after living with this disease for 35 years." "Who the $%^* are you to tell me anything?" "Do you take 13,000 pills a year?" "Do you have to find time to sit in machines for 90 minutes a day?" "Are you running marathons?" "By the looks of your gut, you don't do %$#@ to take care of yourself—so don't tell me what I need to do." "Get the %$#@ out of my room." It may not have been my most charitable moment, but that day, I had reached the end of my patience.

Those are the things I *wanted* to say, but I wasn't ready to unleash my fury on the "dumb kid" doctor. I did kick him out of the room, unable to hide all my interior venom, and instructed my doctor to never send in that idiot again. I even begged my doctor to not unleash that man on anyone else. That felt good for about 30 seconds—then I felt like a jerk. That venom was building up over 30 + years of sitting in a doctor's office, hearing people tell me how to live my life better or else. That was thirty years of being talked AT, and I was tired of it.

On the other hand, the conversations with my primary doctor are awesome. For one, I respect him tremendously as an M.D. Secondly, I just plain and simple like him as a human being. I think we could even have beers and laugh together outside of the exam room. I know I can't expect him to love and care for me as he would his family or friends; that's not what I'm asking for. I simply want others to speak WITH me as, not TO me, as if I'm a machine. I often remind him of the vast array of things he asks me to do that I *am* compliant with. In addition, I think it's obvious I take ownership of my condition. I run marathons, have gained weight, take a lot of medicine, and have stayed out of serious medical trouble under his medical supervision. I owe so much to his thoughtful guidance and support over the years. I actually look forward to seeing him and his staff. As a result of him caring about me, I feel loyalty toward him and want to do well for him, so he can see happy results. I don't just work hard for my wife and myself. Part of my motivation is to make my doctor's hard work worthwhile. I hope our relationship has been as rewarding for him as it has been for me.

When you interact as real people, you can say many things that normally are off the table. He told me not long ago that my "charms" will no longer work on him. What he meant is that my ability to run marathons gave me some leeway in his eyes. When my lung capacity numbers were not improving, he was able to put his foot down in a manner of speaking and let me know that I had to get better. He was able to gently remind me that if I didn't control all aspects of this disease, I could die. Most people think that sounds cruel, but he has permission to talk to me directly, because we've built a trusting relationship. I trust his motivation for telling me something like that straight up, and I take it to heart.

The Long Haul

The most difficult aspect of taking care of oneself is the duration of time in which I have to stay vigilant. This is a *lifetime* thing. It's intriguing that MLB players call a single season "The Grind." These ball players will lament on the day in, day out life of a baseball player. Long hours each day. Months of travel, workouts, practice, and games. Always having to be "on." I'm not bashing these guys for their notion of "the grind." I actually understand what they mean, because I know what it is like to be required to stay on top of one's game every single day. My analogy is imperfect of course, because these athletes get at least a bit of a break each winter and their career is not over a lifetime. My medical condition (and your life for that matter) has no off-season. If I slack off, there *will* be repercussions, and they could be deadly. There are no motivational speakers coming to see me, no "Wiley Veterans" to pump me up, and no grand prize of a World Series to rest my cap on.

Recently, there was a Cardinals player in St. Louis who will undoubtedly go down as one of the greatest baseball players in his generation. What a fun time it was to see him do amazing things with the God-given talents he possesses. I find it very interesting, though, that this great natural talent is surrounded by coaches. He has a hitting coach. He has a fielding coach. He even has a guy who prepares film of his at bats so that when he's between innings, he can immediately correct his swing or anticipate a pitch coming. He has also had a Hall Of Fame manager since the day he came to the pros. When he was a Cardinal, there were a handful of "Hall of Famers" giving him sage advice. Considering all this, is it any surprise that he is as successful as he is, with his abundance of natural talent nurtured by many supportive coaches? It is not a coincidence that he has done well with the qualified mentors he has had.

So why don't *we* have more coaches in life? Do we think we are weak when we ask for advice? Are we too proud to seek help? Do we think we know everything? I don't know why we insist on learning stuff the hard way, but I've learned having a few coaches is a great thing. These can be actual life coaches or just awesome people who have some strength to offer that you simply don't possess yet. Hopefully you're confident enough to receive a tough message every once in a while and take it with humility. Admitting you don't know what you don't know is the first big step. Finding a mentor or coach that can keep you fired up to live well and keep you accountable when you slack is a benefit that cannot be underestimated.

Life's No Guarantee

Not only is living with this challenge a lifetime journey, there are also no guarantees that if I take the medicine and put in the hours of therapy and exercise that all will turn out well. It becomes especially difficult when you are doing everything asked for and more and still land in the hospital.

By the beginning of 2011, after completing nine marathons and nearly twenty half marathons, I had maintained excellent health by normal standards, much less by the measures of this disease. I wanted to keep this going and keep exercise interesting, so it was time to up the ante. In the spirit of keeping the challenge high, I decided to try triathlons. Swimming, biking, and running would also definitely keep me on my toes and keep my body healthy.

To illustrate my point: in March of 2011, I trained for a 70.3 Ironman Triathlon, which consists of 1.2 miles of swimming (in a lake or river) followed by 56 miles of biking and 13.1 miles of running. Each discipline follows the other without resting. During training, I was getting into the best shape of my life. My lungs were clear and my weight was optimal. To keep the weight on during all the required exercise, I was eating at least 4,000 calories a day of the healthiest food I had ever eaten. To keep my body at peak performance, I was very consistent with the various treatments prescribed. I was as compliant as I ever had been and feeling great about being so healthy.

Not even halfway through my training, I developed a minor cold. One Friday, during the day I was feeling a bit fatigued. Thinking it was just from training and a business trip, I reduced my bicycle mileage that day and rested. I was planning on making up the mileage on Sunday. By Saturday morning I had decided to rest from exercise the whole weekend because I could feel something coming on. By Saturday night, the little aches from Friday had developed into a stuffy nose and a bit of coughing. This is how a typical cold starts for me, so I called the doctor and asked for antibiotics. Usually a round of antibiotics will knock out the cold within a few days. By Sunday, my cough was worse than normal and I ached all over. With every breath, I could hear and feel a "rattle" in my lungs. That rattle made me cough with nearly every breath. By the end of Sunday I was so sore from coughing I couldn't sleep. Every muscle in my head, neck, shoulders, back, and torso hurt. I felt like Sonny Liston must have felt in the Muhammad Ali photo I mentioned—totally beat up! I told my wife, Rene, that I was going to call the doctor on Monday morning and give him the report. I told her to brace for a hospital stay because I couldn't remember coughing like that in my life. Sure enough, on Monday I was admitted into the hospital. Late

Monday night, I started running a 103-degree fever. By Tuesday morning I didn't want to eat anything and the cough was not letting up. I'd never been so miserable and I was very disappointed that my training was going to take a serious setback. How crazy was I obsessing about missing training, when my body had a 103-degree fever! Over the next 5 days, I got progressively better. It took some high-potency antibiotics and complete bed rest, but I beat that infection.

The final medical procedure the doctor did for me was to take a Pulmonary Function Test (PFT). This requires blowing into a little machine that measures lung capacity. 100% is obviously optimal. My pulmonary functions had hovered just above 80% for a good decade. This percentage equates to a mild effect from my disease. The resulting figure of this latest PFT, however, was below 65%. In one week, I had lost nearly 15% of my lung function. The worst thing was that there was no culprit. No flu bugs; no pneumonia. No other bug was found in my lungs other than the two bugs I've hosted for years. My diagnosis: my disease was just doing what it does normally.

Without warning, I went from training for a triathlon to a hospital bed, losing significant lung function in the span of one week. One can react in one of two ways here: the first is to throw up your hands, give up, and declare, "See, it doesn't matter what I do." Or, you can refuse to give in to creeping despair and give all you have in order to conquer the physical and mental battle. At least for the time, I was still in conquering mode. I continued with training with a one-week setback, and went on to race the Muncie 70.3 Ironman in July of 2011. I competed in that race with my lung capacity hovering between 65-70% of a normal 42-year-old. The entire year of 2011, I was frustrated at how my disease was greatly affecting my ability to perform physical activities. Even with all my successes, my setbacks of 2011 were a constant reminder that I had no guarantees of health or fitness. My health situation was ever changing, and I couldn't afford to take even one day for granted.

Pushing Forward in 2012

After competing in that 70.3 Ironman and failing to finish, I was all the more frustrated. I could feel the effects of the disease. I was breathing hard at speeds I could previously run comfortably. I was coughing more at slower speeds, during both cycling and running. My frustration and worry were growing, but I continued to work out, knowing that at least I had a better chance of maintaining the lung function I did have. Over that winter, I broke any remaining resistance I had to being compliant. In 2012, I had to reduce my goal of finishing an Ironman to finishing an Olympic Distance Triathlon. Even though that race was half the distance of an Ironman, it was physically crushing for me. I was used to being able to do the most difficult things; not that I was exceptionally good, but I could do them previously and now I could not. It was a struggle to stay motivated, but I stayed focused and worked extra hard to get in shape.

On top of the exercise regimen, I started a new drug which I had previously resisted taking. By June of 2012, I was feeling really good. My swim times were fast again, and running and biking were producing less heavy breathing. In June I had a doctor's appointment scheduled where we would test lung capacity. I was not dreading this appointment because I was doing everything I could and was feeling fine. I would blow into the machine and just hope the results would be at least maintaining last year's results. *Just stay even, don't lose anymore.*

From the breathing test room, I went over to the doctor's office. When the doctor asked if I knew the results, I told him the lab tech said they were all right. The doctor looked shocked! He corrected me and said my results were *awesome*. I had gained back 20% of the lung capacity previously lost. My lung function decline had not only stopped—I was able to gain back some. My lungs showed airflow numbers equal to my 2008 numbers. I couldn't believe it! The hard work and compliance had paid off and my sense of relief was palpable. I had not realized how much mental weight I was carrying over the past few years, especially in 2011 following the hospital stay. I thought the creeping decline of lung function wasn't bothering me all that much. Receiving this news and having a sense of relief wash over me was incredibly rewarding. Compliance can not only help strengthen you for the long haul, but it can produce moments of complete satisfaction in the short term.

Urgency: What It Means

The third most difficult part of taking care of myself, after the challenges of the "long haul" and "no guarantees," is when I don't feel any *urgency* to do so. What urgency am I talking about?

Pain! Without feeling pain, it's easy not to take medicine. In my own instance, if I don't take digestive enzymes I feel discomfort within hours and true pain within a day. Without pills to digest food, my belly gets bloated and sore within 24 hours. Within 48 hours, I develop severe diarrhea. There are immediate and painful consequences when not taking this medicine.

Other medicine I take is more preventative. Insulin is a good example. Unlike the digestive enzymes, which have immediate effects, there are not always alarms the body sends when I mismanage insulin intake. Over time, however, not taking insulin will result in death. Even though I know that death can happen as a result of high blood sugar, it is more difficult to remain vigilant with insulin, because my body isn't "screaming" at me. This is a good example of the need to use sheer willpower to take preventative measures in health. For the times when your body isn't constantly reminding you to take a remedy—I've found the voice of a loved one is a good substitute.

"Big Boy Pants"

I've also found that if I have a goal to focus on that requires good health, it is easier to be positive about taking all my medicine. For me, the focus is running better, biking longer, and not drowning in a pool because I had a blood sugar crash. I want to be a better athlete, so I take medicine to be stronger. I also do it for my wife. I want to be with her for a long time. I do it for my parents because they worked very hard for me throughout my childhood. I do it for other families with my condition because it is uplifting to see an older person with my condition do so well in life.

My final thought on this whole compliance issue: the more you implement changes to take care of yourself, the more you "own" your life. By definition, to *own* something means to have power or mastery over something. How can I have power and mastery over a genetic disease that I had no influence over, which will do what it does, sometimes regardless of my actions? While I can't control what happens around me or even control what my body will do, I can still have power over the disease. I own what I do everyday, and I own my thoughts. Either I can own the failure to take medicine, or I can own taking the medicine. If I take the medicine and exercise as I'm advised, I can have mastery over the reaction to bad news. In the past 13 years, the news has not always been good for me, but I am equipped with the comfort of knowing that I work hard at taking care of my body and I don't have regrets. If I was completely slacking on *compliance* all those years and got the same bad news, I think I would be full of regret. Being full of regret and letting your circumstance dictate who you are and how you feel means you are being owned, and no one enjoys that feeling. Your focus, your reason for compliance, can be ANYTHING that drives you to WANT to take the medicine. Choose something to strive for!

With all that medicine, all that therapy, and all the uncertainty come a great battle. To be alone in that battle is unimaginable for me. I have been fortunate to have a great many people at my side. The sheer number of people and the timing with which they come into my life has been inexplicable to me for years. Without them, my life would be much harder. I want to thank them by telling their stories.

Chapter 4

MOM AND DAD

*"When I was a kid my parents moved a lot,
but I always found them."*

Rodney Dangerfield, American comedian

Naturally, the beginning of my life starts with my parents. I love and respect them greatly. What I admire the most about them is the love they have always brought to my life. No matter what was going on or what I did to deserve their anger or frustration, they loved me. While I can't recall lots of specific advice they have given, the life they've lived is the greatest way they "preached" to me and my brothers—by their good example. Their ability to be a team for over 50 years and raise four levelheaded, successful human beings—and have so many friends I can't count—is tribute enough to who they are. I have to let you in on who Jack and Pat are, because it's their unique personalities that were so important to my life. They formed the person I am today.

Mom (Pat)

My mom is one tough woman, and family has always been at the center of her life. There is nothing more important to her than being surrounded by her boys and our families. She missed us greatly when we were grown and scattered to the four winds chasing careers. Mom's desire for a loving family came from an uncommon place. I can't tell you everything about her early life, because that is a whole book in and of itself, so here is the quick summary: she was adopted into a wonderful little family. Her father was doting and her mother was loving. They were financially stable and lived a nice life in a working-class neighborhood in St. Louis. Mom has a photo album filled with pictures and captions written by her father. There are countless pictures taken at her birthdays, First Communion, Christmas, Easter, and other celebrations. Cute captions were written telling us about those special days and revealing the loving nature of my maternal grandfather. My mother's happy life changed when her adopted mother passed away when Pat was 14. Her mother had been sick, so it wasn't a great surprise, but nonetheless it was traumatic. Her father struggled immensely and did not handle it well. As her father began to drink heavily, my mother lost the attentive father figure she was accustomed to. At the very same time, she lost a sister. Her sister was a foster child, but had lived with the family for many years and was considered a permanent part of the family. The foster care system in that day did not allow a single male to have a female in the household, so her sister was pulled from them. I can't imagine losing your spouse and daughter in this tragic manner.

Amidst his despair, her father turned to another woman for comfort. Unfortunately for my mom, this new stepmother was no peach. In fact, she hated my mother. This series of events affected my mother profoundly. If this would have happened a few years before or a few years later, the effects might not have been as bad. This all happened in my mother's most formative years as a young teenager. This change in her life is one of the reasons a tight-knit family is so very important to her. I also believe this is why she developed such a tough-minded will. She was determined to have the stable, loving family life that was taken from her as a teenager.

Wrestle Royale

Later in her life, my mother had her hands full with four boys who were rather rambunctious. By the time we were in high school, we were taller and stronger than her. Somehow she managed to keep the house down to a mild roar, and when we got too rambunctious, she would find ways to end the shenanigans. When we were teenagers we called her "Momma Hogan." For those that don't remember, there was a famous wrestler in the 1980's whose name was Hulk Hogan. He was a gigantic man with bulging muscles and his big body matched his big personality. My mother is all of 5'2" and I believe she could take down Hulk Hogan. She was that strong and determined. In spite of her toughness, "Momma Hogan" is an incredibly loving mother. All she ever wanted was for her boys to love one another, be happy in their lives, and be good men. While we brothers were rambunctious and combative, we did spend a great deal of peaceful time together as well. When mom went back to work and it was summertime, we were basically around each other 24/7. I can't speak for my brothers, but for myself, I really liked having brothers growing up. Getting in each other's way was inevitable, but I was and still am proud to have them as siblings. Mom helped us realize what that meant and the greatest lesson we took from her was that we were brothers and that we had a special bond. No matter what we disagree on, we are brothers and when the "stuff hits the fan" we will stand with one another.

Dad (Jack)

My dad is the guy that everybody likes. He has three great talents that endear him to everyone: one, he can spin a story like nobody else (and he's got loads of stories). Two, he knows every random, trivial piece of information you'll ever want to know. As a result of these talents, he acquired two nicknames: "Turbo Tongue" and "Cliffy." (Do you remember Cliff Claven from the TV show *Cheers*? Yes, the mailman who knew everything.) I'll have to admit I learned quite a bit from Dad, and he's not annoying like Cliffy was. Three, he can make a personal connection to you and loves trying to figure it out. Do you know about the game *Seven Degrees of Kevin Bacon*? The main gist of the game is that, within seven people, Kevin Bacon has acted in a movie with everyone in Hollywood. With the same concept as the Kevin Bacon game, my dad knows you. I've never seen it fail. It's fun to watch him work to find the connections between people and I learned to do that as well. It is an amazing way to get to know people.

He's not just the guy that everybody likes because he tells a great story. He would also do anything for you, and everybody knows it. Dad was also a great example to his sons to strive for achievement. Overall, his outward message as we were growing up was to be good and do right by others. Work hard at school and work hard in your career. Seems like a simple message, and it is. Most importantly, his actions back up those words. Early in his career, Dad rose through the ranks at a very respectable company. He had been working hard for a promotion, so when his boss called him in and awarded my father the promotion, he was overjoyed. There was a caveat to this promotion, however. The boss told him that this was his last promotion, as my father did not have a college degree. The next promotions were to executive-level jobs, and those required formal education. The promotion he had just received was a good job with more than acceptable income. Simply keeping this level of responsibility and income would have kept life comfortable for my father.

Apparently, Mom and Dad had bigger goals. After Dad came home that night, Mom and Dad talked. It happened that Grandma and Grandpa Burke were also there, and all were excited. When Dad recounted what the boss had said about his future, a plan was hatched. Dad was going to get a college degree. He would be the first in his family to do so. I mention my grandparents because they were very supportive in this decision. Grandpa was very proud of my dad and was 100% behind this new goal. Although my grandfather might not have been an eloquent speaker, his words had purpose, and when he said, "Boy, go get you one of those" (a degree), my father knew *everyone* was behind him.

Somehow, in the midst of raising four boys, working a regular full time job, getting to soccer games, and spending time with us, he earned his college degree. Dad would be promoted further until he was an executive in charge of a division. Unfortunately for us boys, when we were in college and perhaps struggling with our own grades or juggling part-time work and school, there was simply no excuse for us! I can't tell you how many times I heard "Your father got straight A's while working a job and raising you fools!" This is not something you want to hear when you're young, but I can't think of many better examples than Dad. That is his personality. He was always helping to organize something and putting in "sweat equity." He helped build soccer fields for church. He assisted the other fathers in coordinating the picnics and athletic association. He helped local nuns when they needed help. He coached soccer and started the first soccer club in our area.

Dad got the fun part. Everybody knew him and he received the promotions and saw projects through to completion. He got the glory, but without Mom behind him, none of it would have happened. She ran the Burke Operation at home, and that allowed Dad to be out and doing such things. Her part was just as critical as Dad's; plus, she had to deal with the "monkeys" at home. (God bless her!) Mom and Dad were a team in all of this. They made a plan together and sometimes that plan went as scheduled. Many times, though, their plan went all to pieces and they had to adjust things. Sometimes they didn't have a plan but made things work anyway. Raising four boys, one with a chronic illness, was a true challenge but they rose to every occasion. Keeping life normal for a kid who would be constantly seeing his short life expectancy right before his eyes would require toughness, planning, adjusting, humor, love, and drive. All these things could be seen in my parent's marriage as I was growing up. With Mom's tough spirit and love of family and Dad's positive outlook on all things, they seemed an ideal pair to tackle the lifelong challenge coming their way.

The Good Life

There is not much in this world that conjures up an image of "the good life" more than a family. Think of high school sweethearts getting married, having three healthy sons, a dog, a nice little house, financial stability, a good future, and a large extended family all living close. Is this Stepford? The only thing that would be better is another child. Hopefully this time it would be a girl. Mom wanted a girl; as a matter of fact, each of the first three boys were assigned a girl's name, Maureen. Well, Maureen wasn't to be. The fourth child was another baby boy: me. Another healthy and rambunctious male.

My arrival necessitated moving to a larger house. The house and neighborhood we moved into were perfect for four growing boys. There were a multitude of kids and big backyards. There were enough children that backyard games of all sorts could be formed in an instant. Our home had a big, flat yard, and it quickly became the baseball diamond, football field, and general gathering place for the entire neighborhood. Our basement was large and unfinished, so it became the hockey rink during winter. Can you imagine a dozen kids on metal roller skates playing hockey in a basement? There was even a "checking wall" made of flexible paneling where the unsuspecting players were ruthlessly thrust mid-skate. Only the occasional loud "DONG" would bring my father downstairs to check on us. The "DONGGGGG" indicated that somebody had run into a metal support pole. (Don't worry, nobody died.) It was awesome! There was always a house full of wild boys. All was perfect—almost.

(The Gross Part)

What is that green stuff that he coughs up, and for "Cripes" sake, what is in his diaper?! "Cripes" was my mother's way of not taking the Lord's name in vain. (I wonder if it is a St. Louis thing, because in all the other places I've lived, I've never heard that phrase said.) Anyhow, at about six weeks old, I developed a persistent cough. By persistent I mean non-stop. Not only was I coughing, but what was coming up was truly disgusting. Let's take a moment to describe the mucus. You know that stuff you cough up when you have a really nasty cold or the flu? Green and thick. The kind of stuff that sticks to whatever you spit it on. Imagine that sticky stuff in your lungs all the time. This is what their infant was coughing up. Think back to the last time you were really sick and coughing. From the incessant coughing, your head hurts, your neck hurts, throat hurts, and back muscles hurt from all the convulsions. Now think what all that coughing must do to an infant's body. With all that crying, my mother thought the neighbors would call the police because there was some kind of abuse going on. When the coughing got really bad and was accompanied by a fever, I would be taken to the hospital. The diagnosis was consistently pneumonia. I was taken to the hospital three times before I was a year old, each time with pneumonia.

The doctors were not at all sure what the source of all the infections was. I can't imagine the fear and frustration that a mother and father must feel to have no control over their baby's health. How helpless must it be to listen to your baby cry in pain? In addition to the disgusting green mucus, my bowel movements were not normal. I was experiencing chronic diarrhea, accompanied by quite a bit of chronic stomach pain. Throughout the months of infections and diarrhea, our family doctor was experimenting and trying to pinpoint a diagnosis. The first thing he tried was a room humidifier running throughout the night. The humidifier would shoot mist at my face and hopefully clear up the lungs. At the same time, the doctor was testing for allergies. The only way to thoroughly do that was to experiment with food and switching up my diet constantly.

All of this was very time-consuming and my mom was busy trying to raise four boys, so friends and family began to pitch in.

The Extended Family

Family pitched in where they could and settled into their roles. Uncle John, who is an awesome chef, would make rice cakes and other recipes in the hopes of isolating a food allergy. Grandma and Grandpa were always around to help. Grandpa's self-appointed role was to drive the 45 minutes one way into the city and pick up various medicines for my vaporizer. He also happened to be the only other person I would go to, aside from my mom. That is particularly strange because he was a tall, scary-looking guy. I suppose our children know us best sometimes; only later in life would I hear of all the stories about how my grandfather was a big softie at heart.

Aunt Sis

My mom's special helper in life was my Aunt Sis. Aunt Sis was my father's sister and a widow who never had children of her own. The nieces and nephews were her babies, and she spoiled us rotten. Sis was so much more than an aunt. She was at every baptism, every birthday, graduation, and family vacation. Aside from my father, she was the greatest source of support for my mom. In some ways she was an even greater support than my father, because Aunt Sis was the older sister my mom never truly had. Since she was single and had no children, Sis was always available to help. She was not only available, but made sure it was never a question that she would be there when help was needed. My mother felt more relaxed when Sis was around. She was a shoulder to lean on; she was a happy, witty, and very fun-loving woman. She never wanted or asked for anything in return. It seemed Sis was on earth to be there for everyone.

Aunt Sis did get "payback," although she never asked for anything. This payback was probably not what she would have preferred, and of course it came from me. When I was 4 or so years old my mom had to have surgery. The extended family pitched in and we boys went to various aunt and uncles' houses for a week. Aunt Sis got saddled with me. Apparently, I didn't like what she was telling me to do one day. In a huff I disappeared into her bedroom. As I emerged from the bedroom, I was dragging her suitcase behind me. Demanding that she leave and declaring to the world "I don't like you," I proceeded to drop the suitcase at her feet.

Our conflict was resolved in the fashion in which all conflicts with her were resolved: Aunt Sis turned to humor and love. First she made me put the suitcase back, and while I was sulking, she hugged and kissed me until I couldn't resist giggling. All this culminated in a treat (probably chocolate chip cookies or one of the best hamburgers that this planet has ever seen). To this day, my mother loves to tell that story.

When Sis died, my cousin John shared the greatest compliment Sis could have received. He said everyone was convinced that they were her favorite. Our family, especially my mother, was influenced tremendously by her love. She was my mom's angel; she took care of Grandma and Grandpa Burke in their old age, and loved us all as her own. I wonder if she really realized how important she was.

The Final Verdict

The family was pulling together, but the doctors were no closer to figuring things out. There was an ongoing effort of changes in my diet trying to eliminate the problem. Near my 14th month of life, I was once again sick. Previous infections sounded the same, so Mom and Dad were expecting another hospital visit. I was now underweight for my age due to my digestion issues, so things were getting critical. The family practitioner must have been incredibly frustrated. No matter what he tried, the source of my problems was eluding him. Back at the doctor with another infection, Mom was bracing for the hospital. Finally the light bulb went off. The doctor put together the coughing, the thick mucus, the pneumonia, the diarrhea, AND lack of allergies.

He urged my parents: he wanted me to go to a well-known pediatric specialist the very next day. No time was to be wasted. He suggested to my parents that I was exhibiting the symptoms of a serious childhood disease. That night, my mom looked up the symptoms. (Remember, there was no Internet, so she tracked down a medical book.) Upon reading the signs of this disease, she decided that I was in fact showing its classic symptoms. At that point she knew; Dad, however, wanted confirmation. Before the advent of genetic testing, the suspect disease was confirmed with a sweat test. Patients with this disease have an unusually high salt content in their sweat, so that was the major indicator. The next day my sweat test was positive, and the day after that the pediatric hospital confirmed a second sweat test.

The clinical description of the disease sounds like this: *An inherited chronic disease that affects the lungs and digestive system. It produces thick, sticky mucus that clogs the lungs, leads to life-threatening lung infections, and obstructs the pancreas. It also stops natural enzymes from absorbing food. The life expectancy is five years. The baby will experience very salty-tasting skin, persistent coughing, frequent lung infections, wheezing or shortness of breath, poor growth, and frequent greasy stools or difficulty with bowel movements.*

Unless you're a robot, the following thoughts would flood your mind: your baby will suffer tremendous pain from chronic pneumonia and diarrhea. Your baby will die before getting to kindergarten. Your child will never go to school, play soccer, or have his First Communion. He will not graduate from high school or college, nor grow old enough to have a family of his own. And you, Mom and Dad, will have a giant hole in your heart.

I'd like you to stop for a moment and take that in. As a parent, your hope of hopes is to find out what is wrong with your child. If you only knew what the problem was, you could do something about it. Now, however, you almost wish you didn't know because the outlook is so devastating.

Reaction

My mother was very worried thinking of how desperate the situation was. Dad reacted differently; like a lot of people, he wanted to know what to do. Underneath the desire to do something, Dad feared something many of us fear. Dad has told me that his worst nightmare is the image of one of us boys falling off a cliff and being unable to grab us in time. Deep down, he was worried about not being able to do what needed to be done to fix this. It was horrible for him to be a helpless bystander. In typical "Jack and Pat" fashion, they didn't get stuck in those negative thoughts—they set to work learning how they could handle this new challenge.

The doctors had a few things they could try. There were antibiotics to help the lung infections and there were digestive enzymes that could be mixed with food to optimize digestion. My mom and dad now had at least something to do. With antibiotics, the pneumonia stopped and didn't return. The coughing was significantly reduced. With the enzymes, the diarrhea stopped, and although I was smaller than normal I began to gain weight. Most importantly of all, I *stopped crying.* That meant I was no longer in constant pain; there were hope and solid results to hold onto.

Patience

I keep saying how tough my mother is. You would have to be not only strong, but also patient when dealing with doctors, hospitals, insurance companies, and the quarterly visits to the specialty clinic. Part of the regimen of care was to visit the clinic every 3 months. No matter what was going on in Mom and Dad's lives, a clinic appointment was never missed. Now, this isn't just any ordinary trip to the doctor. I want to put this into perspective, so I'll explain this routine my mom had to follow.

Take off work early. Pick up Michael from school just before lunch. Take him out for a "special" lunch at Burger Chef to make the day easier. Drive 40 minutes to downtown St. Louis. Wait to be registered. Register. Go to x-ray lab. Wait at x-ray lab. Get x-rays done. Go to lab for sputum culture. Wait at lab. Watch as son is gagged and coughs uncontrollably because technicians have stuck a very long Q-tip down his throat. Wait for flu shot. Get flu shot. Let squirming son enjoy a sucker. Wait for doctor. See doctor and get an update. Go to pharmacy to get prescriptions. Wait in line at pharmacy. Get prescriptions and make the drive back home—now in the middle of rush hour traffic.

The required waiting was excruciating. This caused a single visit to the doctor to be a day-long event and surely an exercise in patience. Fortunately, once I started taking the medicine, my checkups were not producing more bad news.

One Brave Momma

Back in the "olden days," all families would go to a doctor's clinic on the same day. There was only one specialist doctor who knew anything about the disease, so that is who you saw. On most visits, there would be 4 to 6 families in the clinic, and Mom would get to know them a bit. In one respect, they could give my mom someone to talk to. In another respect, it was very difficult. More times than she would like to experience, a family would not return. It's not difficult to deduce what had happened. There was no other specialty clinic within 100 miles. This disease was devastating to children. Adding to the stress, there was only one young adult that my mother had ever seen at this clinic. From all this you could easily assume that individual families did not return because the child had died, but you surely were not going to talk about that with the other moms. Many times when the families didn't return, she would be conflicted with differing emotions. How could she be so happy that Michael was so "healthy" while other kids were dying? When people are being wimpy, they are told to "man up." But I think they should say "momma up." To my mom's credit, I can't remember these visits being anything other than getting a day off school. (Other than the visits that I was getting a flu shot, because I was always convinced that was the end of the world!)

Moving On and Letting Go — For the Most Part

Germs are bad. Germs make normal children sick. Germs kill kids with my condition. My parents were unsure about what to do when it came to me playing with my older brothers and the neighborhood kids. What the doctors were advising is to try and keep Michael away from germs when possible. Did that mean Michael would need to live in a bubble? Mom and Dad were struggling with these questions when a critical moment happened.

As I mentioned previously, our yard was big and flat and perfect for all sorts of sports. One winter day, a football game was being played in the Burke backyard. As Dad recalls, it really wasn't a football game as much as it was a chaotic melee of running and tackling. There could have been up to 15 kids yelling, tumbling, and beating on each other. All my brothers were out there as well as my buddies from the neighborhood. Keep in mind—this is when kids of all ages played together and there was no mercy for the littler guys. It was a grand winter slugfest that all the boys wanted to get in on. There would be bloody noses, black eyes and bruised muscles, all of which would provide bragging rights when the game was over.

I was inside, standing at the patio door, looking through the glass at the fun going on outside. My father was watching me watch the other boys. He was struggling to decide if I should be out there or not. He worried about the cold day. He worried about his "sick" boy getting hurt. He worried about the germs that all those boys were carrying. Mostly, he worried that I was doomed to a life of exclusion. Watching me watching them, Dad remembered the words of the doctor: "Keep Michael active. I want Michael to do whatever his brothers do."

Not able to take it anymore, Dad quietly asked my mom to get me ready to go outside. Like a racehorse at the starting gate, I shot outside when Dad opened the door. Even before I reached the pile of players, one of the neighbor kids took me out. Apparently it was a pretty good hit, as I was knocked off my feet. Dad was watching all this unfold with a white-knuckle grip on the door handle. Just as he was about to come and rescue me, I got up, dusted myself off, and headed into the fray for more action. My father is often asked what he did after that moment. Dad's simple response was, "I turned away and never watched again." Dad knew that if he watched, he would never let me be a normal kid. From that point on, Mom and Dad let me do what normal kids did. Sometimes the best medicine is to simply live a normal life.

Through the coming years, though, I gave them plenty to worry about. They watched from a distance with "one hand on the door" in case I didn't get up and dust myself off. But they never intruded.

Chapter 5

THE BROTHERS NOT SO GRIM

*"I can do things you cannot. You can do things
I cannot. Together we can do great things."*

Mother Teresa

Thank God we humans are different. Perhaps life would be easier if everyone thought just like me, but I suppose boredom would kick in if that were the case. More importantly, I would miss seeing fresh perspectives on life. I used to believe people were a big disappointment because they couldn't handle what I needed regarding life with a chronic illness. I also thought people didn't care because they didn't react or respond in the ways that I wanted them to. At some point, the realization set in that I shouldn't be angry or disappointed with people. I learned that people have different approaches to life and different strengths. If you can find out what they are best at, you can build a support system with many different strengths. Some will be warm and affectionate. Others will be analytical and levelheaded. Some will go out of their way to let you know they will help. Others will quietly work magic without your ever knowing. I find it rare indeed that you will find someone that genuinely doesn't care.

After that fateful day of backyard football, my parents were able to let go of a great deal of their fear. They didn't feel the need to be literally watching over me. They took a leap of courage to allow me to be a regular kid. I'm sure they experienced a great deal of trepidation, but they would get help protecting me from a source they most likely didn't expect. I don't think they ever counted on the vital role of my older brothers.

If I were going to be brutally honest, I would more accurately describe my siblings not as "brothers" but as "tortures!" The torture chambers of the Medieval and Dark Ages had nothing on my brothers. You would think that I would catch some slack having a life-threatening disease, but that was only wishful thinking.

I've told stories to many people about what life was like in a house with four boys. When I recount our adventures of wrestling matches turned real fights, name-calling, "loogie-drooling," and general rowdiness, I get two reactions. The first is horror, which comes from people who didn't have brothers. They look at me with terror in their eyes, wondering how we are alive, much less how we could care for one another. They also wonder how horrid my parents must have been for letting these things happen. The second reaction is complete understanding and camaraderie, which comes from people who also grew up in a house full of boys. Their reaction is "sounds about right." Then I get their own stories about shooting each other with BB guns, bottle-rocket fights, and regular drowning attempts at the pool. Yep, sounds right!

So, how could these seemingly horrific older brothers step into a healthy role for my parents? My big brothers thought something like this: I myself can beat the hell out of Mike, but you better watch yourself because he's MY little brother. My parents encouraged us to love one another, of course. There was a little statue on my oldest brother's nightstand. It was a big kid

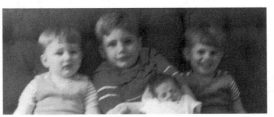

Left to right: Tom, Jack, Matt, and baby brother Mike

carrying a little kid piggyback style. The caption underneath read, "He ain't heavy, he's my brother." I can remember one particular story of how we brothers stuck together. Again, this is probably appalling to families without brothers—but it makes me laugh. We were scrapping with the neighbor boys one day; there were two of them and four of us. You can already see where I'm going. It started with me and the youngest of their family. As boys did back in the day, we started fighting. Being the smallest, I was taking quite a beating. In stepped my brother Tom. Now Tom is two years older than I was and the boy who I was scrapping with, so the tide of battle turned. Coming to my opponent Derek's rescue was his older brother, Jason. As Jason was punching on Tom, in stepped my brother Matt, who was a year older than Jason. That pretty well ended the brawl, as Matt and Tom were too much for Jason by himself. Just when things were getting pretty bad, my father and Jason and Derek's father came out to see what the commotion was about. As Derek and Jason's father saw immediately that his boys were outnumbered, he expressed how unfair this situation was. My dad responded by saying "You should have had more sons." I don't know whether that was right or wrong for my dad to say, but everyone knew that if you messed with one Burke boy, you got them all.

In defense of my dad, that line he said to the other father wasn't what we boys heard. Believe me, we were given an earful for fighting and ganging up on the neighbors. I'm glad to say we still see these neighbors from time to time and we can now laugh and reminisce about the "good ol' days."

There was also something instinctual about my older siblings protecting their little brother. Without it really being said out loud, the boys took care of me. Only when we got older did I appreciate that. The very brothers that gave me countless thrashings became important role models and advice givers, and would always look out for their little brother.

Biggest Brother (Jack)

Jack was instrumental in my life, especially in helping with the fight with my disease. As a teenager, I was coming to grips with my short life expectancy. Jack was quite a bit older than I was, so when I was in high school he was already out of college and working. As a result, he was mature enough to listen to a 16-year-old kid working out his feelings. He lived on his own, which meant I could escape Mom and Dad's house and hang out with my cool older brother. I really admired him because he was adventurous. In high school he was allowed to go away for the summer to work. During college undergraduate work, he worked in Wyoming, which seemed so far away to a kid like myself. When he was earning his masters degree, he was in Siberia for a summer—250 miles inside the Arctic Circle, living in a giant tin shed with a bunch of Russians. That was the coolest thing I'd ever heard of.

One summer, Jack was home from college and I was complaining that I had never been to South Dakota. The whole family had gone on a big vacation out west before I was born. The Black Hills and Yellowstone were a major part of their trip, and I didn't get to go. After hearing their stories, I romanticized the West and always wanted to go to the states my brothers had visited. I think I just had the same adventurous spirit as Jack did, and he empathized with my desire to see great sights. It was that or he was tired of hearing my complaining—he told Mom and Dad he was going to take me to South Dakota. So we got in the car and headed west. Just my big brother and me.

On the first day, we drove from St. Louis to Onawa, Iowa. We camped in a tent next to the Missouri River. There is nothing special about Onawa, Iowa, except that I have a memory with my brother that will last forever. We had a grand adventure. Funny thing about the whole trip is that I remember our dinner that first night. Jack was a good cook, but apparently we forgot to pack camping-appropriate food. In our ravenous state, we improvised and made chili. Of course we had forgotten chili beans, so we had to improvise with baked beans. You know— pork and beans. It was the most horrible meal I've had, and the best meal at the same time! It always makes me laugh whenever I think about it. We drove to Yankton, South Dakota, which was barely across the state line, turned around, and drove right back home. What a memorable adventure for a 14-year-old kid.

Years later, when it was time for me to go away to college, Mom and Dad were nervous; they were wondering if I would take care of myself. They would soon be put at ease, because Jack told them he was going back to school for his master's degree, and he would be going to the University of Missouri at Columbia—the same place I was headed. So Jack and I had another adventure together. Having my brother as my roommate my first year away, I could not have had it any better. Not only did I have the companionship of my older brother, but he served as a safety net as well. At the time I didn't really think of it that way, and didn't appreciate it as a 20-year-old kid. Looking back, however, I realize what a unique and fortunate situation it was to have my brother at college with me. Mom and Dad took great comfort knowing Jack was right there.

Second-Biggest Brother (Matt)

It was fun in high school because when I was a freshman, Matt was a senior. It was nice to walk down the halls and not get abused by the seniors, because my brother was one of their own. Having attended a small grade school and high school, everybody knew everybody. Matt was a popular guy. Smart. Good looking. Athletic. Outgoing. (Don't you hate him already?) That made life easy on me, because before I even arrived in high school, I was already known as "Little Burke." Being small for my age could have resulted in some rough times in high school, but I guess Matt paved the way for me. Having upperclassmen not only know about you, but know you *well* was awesome. Some of those guys had already been hanging around our house for years.

Matt was always good for bringing humor to life. I can remember one time when I was bummed out about not being able to have children. This is a side effect of my condition, and I was focusing on it with a lot of sadness. As I expressed my disappointment about that aspect of my life, he offered a little nugget of humor. It was the kind of advice only a brother can give a brother (and rather indecent), so I can't really repeat it. While wildly inappropriate, his comment made me laugh. That moment allowed me to divert from the seriousness of the moment and have a loosening laugh. Sometimes you just need somebody to snap you out of negative thoughts, and levity can do that in a caring and creative way.

As it happened, Matt could not only provide some humor, but he ended up giving me a job when I graduated from college. I thought I would be able to just cruise along, since my "bro" was my boss. I didn't anticipate his treating me like everyone else. It may sound harsh to some, but he "wrote me up" about six months into the job. I started off great, then got comfortable and started to slack a bit. He sat me down for a serious talk, and he let me know that my work results and work ethic were not good enough. He expressed that if this were to continue, he would actually have to discipline me. I was shocked and a little angry with him for daring to say that I wasn't perfect. The honesty he provided that day was a real wake up call. I thought: if my own brother can write me up, what will a stranger be willing to do? From that day on, I never received discipline from an employer. The experience I gained from Matt's leadership and knowledge has helped me in every job I've had.

Third-Biggest Brother (Tom)

My brother closest in age is Tom. My fondest memories of Tom are the times I asked him to help me solve a problem. Whether it's a business or personal dilemma, he will provide the encouragement or perspective needed. What's interesting is that he never gives advice; he simply asks questions. In the end, he helps people to understand that they already have the best answers, and he simply draws them out. I suppose that is why he is a great leader. He knows how to help people think their own problems through.

Our family is full of adventure; certainly a trait we got from our father. With this love of adventure in mind, Tom treated me to a college graduation present that changed my life. He took me out to Colorado and we fit in so many memorable adventures. In the span of a week, we mountain biked, white-water rafted, hiked, and snow skied. I was so enthralled by the fact that one day I could raft Class IV rapids on the Arkansas River, and the next day ski the tallest resort slope in Colorado. *In May!*

Almost every story about me and my brothers involves something funny or embarrassing. Unfortunately, what I have to tell you next involves both. The first night in Colorado, we camped in the most beautiful spot. We were "up the mountain" from Colorado Springs, 10 or 15 miles west of the little town of Woodland Park. Our camping spot was very primitive. (That meant there was no electricity or running water.) We were camped in a small creek valley with nobody else in sight. The creek was no more than a few feet wide, but had carved a beautiful valley. As we turned off the paved road onto a dirt road, the valley full of tall grass lay before us. This dirt road wound through the grass valley and turned toward the "V" where the valley disappeared into the mountains. As we crossed the creek over a small bridge, we could see the tiny creek making its way across the valley floor like a snake. The road began a small climb, rising 20 or so feet above the creek. When the road ended, we were looking down a small rise at our campsite. The only indication that it was a campsite was the small, numbered wood stake next to the road and the coals left over from a previous campfire. We hauled our gear from the car and set up.

Because this was the first time either of us had camped in the mountains, we were a bit unprepared for how cold it might get overnight. We were so exhausted from a 16-hour overnight drive and a full day of activity that we passed out in our tent. About halfway through the night, I caught an elbow to my ribs. Along with the elbow, Tom urgently said "get off me." All I know is that when he woke me up, I was freezing. Apparently I got a little too close for comfort and "spooned" up against him in the night. Spooning your brother is not cool. In my defense, Tom was quite cold too, so at least I was justified in my action. We put on another layer of clothing, rearranged the sleeping bags and blankets, and all was good.

For the next several days, we mountain biked and camped, working our way up Highway 24 along the Collegiate Peaks into Summit County. We had no idea what we were doing, and it was tremendously exciting. The extent of our preparation was buying a back road map of the counties we were in, so we could bike the trails with some guidance. We would bike half the day, going uphill and then returning downhill with our hair on fire, reaching the bottom in an hour. I had never seen country like this before; I was mesmerized by the beauty of the scenery and extremely happy that I could do so many different exciting things.

I fell in love with Colorado and, just a few years out of college, I moved to Denver so I could be near the adventure that could only be found in the mountains. While living in Colorado, I grew up. I was able to begin focusing on living with this disease on my own terms. I gained the inner strength to live independently and not have to rely on a crutch. I'm sure that wasn't Tom's intention, but many times we will never know the long-reaching implications of the things we do for others.

(After my mother reads this, she will now have someone to blame for her baby boy moving so far from home. Sorry, Tom!)

In this way, our family handled life with my disease. Nothing special was ever made of my condition. I did what the other boys did. My brothers' only approach to life with a chronic illness was an added instinct to protect me—nobody could mess with Mike. This inward sense of protection rubbed off on their friends as well. I was "Little Burke," and there were plenty of big dudes looking out for me. I can't think of a better way to go through high school. I drove to and from school with my brothers every day. I saw them in the halls, at lunch, and on the playing fields. Their girlfriends (who were all gorgeous) would say hello and give me embarrassing hugs in the hallways. Yes, "Little Burke" had it good. They took me to parties, bought me beer, let me visit them when they were in college, and of course Jack invited me into his life when we attended college together. I admire them tremendously for their business success *and* their family success. Their children and wives have great dads and partners who would do anything to ensure their well-being.

I've asked them repeatedly how living with a sibling suffering from a chronic and potentially fatal disease affected their lives. No matter how much prodding I do, I can't get them to say anything dramatic. Their lives were unaffected by my disease, other than watching me take a bunch of medicine and go to the doctor a lot; and I was to be protected like the other brothers. Their stoicism is great testament to my parents, but if you're looking for drama, my brothers may disappoint you. I'm lucky to have three older brothers who helped me, and continue to help me, through a life with unknown challenges. They helped to keep a difficult life fun, adventurous, and focused on the good stuff.

Chapter 6

MID-LIFE CRISIS

"At every crisis in one's life, it is absolute salvation to have some sympathetic friend to whom you can think aloud without restraint or misgiving."

Woodrow Wilson, 28th President

So, I'm 44 and writing about a mid-life crisis. One might think this is a recent event, but in reality it happened many years ago. My understanding of a mid-life crisis is this: as a result of a significant life event, we reevaluate our priorities or goals. Simple enough, don't you think? It seems to me that we suddenly realize what we have or have not done in our life, and on top of that, we also realize that we don't have much time left. We are staring at mortality. The middle-aged person realizes their life is half over, feels they haven't accomplished enough, and then feels compelled to do something about it. We laugh at the image of a 45-year-old bald man buying a sports car, getting a ridiculous hairpiece and new clothes, and spending a weekend in Vegas (and the stories of that trip will never leave Vegas!).

Along the way, the middle-aged adventurer often makes terrible decisions based on selfish motives. He does this all in an attempt to avoid the reality of not accomplishing anything of value in life. In a way, this is what I experienced at age 16. As a friend has noted, my experience was more like an end-of-life crisis than a mid-life crisis.

Whatever you want to call it, this is what I experienced during my sophomore year of high school. I remember sitting in my high school parking lot, in my parents' Chevy Citation. What a God-awful car—right up there with my best friend's lime-green Maverick. My friend Katrina and I were "cruising" after a basketball game, looking for friends to hang with. You don't so much "cruise" in a Chevy Citation as "clunk," but nevertheless we were enjoying ourselves out on the town. Katrina was a great friend, and for some reason I had to get the weight of living with this disease off my chest. I had just passed my 16th birthday, and I was very upset that my life expectancy was age 18. As a result of living with this brief life expectancy, I evaluated my life and what it meant to be living with a disease that gave my body a very short expiration date.

As I was growing up, my parents didn't make a big deal about life with this disease, so it wasn't upsetting to me. Quite frankly, they didn't make anything of it. My brothers didn't make anything of it. All my siblings considered me a "pain in the behind" little brother and nothing more. My best friends rarely asked questions about my disease. You would think with all the medicines and doctors' trips and therapies, *somebody* would have made a big deal about it. Not so. I am thankful that life was kept simple for as long as it was. After all, what is a parent to do? Point out the fact that you have a life-threatening disease? And then point out that there isn't much you can do about it?

In the days leading up to my sixteenth birthday, I was becoming more and more aware that I was living with a fatal disease. In the previous couple of summers, I had spent a week in the hospital for a "tune up". The purpose of this tune up was to flush out as many germs as possible from my body and put some weight on my bones. While in the hospital, I had run across other patients who were not doing so well. Some of these kids spent time in the hospital quite often, and not just for a tune up. They were truly sick. In a deeper way, I started to think about why I was taking thousands of pills and needing all these treatments. Although my friends didn't make a commotion about things, they did occasionally ask questions. They were curious about why I was in the hospital when I seemed so normal. (Well, at least physically normal.) I was also a sophomore in high school, which meant that I was starting to make new friends and eventually needing to explain to them what was going on. While I didn't tell them many details—I didn't want to stand out as "different"—I did think about the subject quite a bit.

I really began pondering what this whole thing *meant*. I went to the library to find more information about the disease. There was no Internet or social media at the time, so I really had to make an effort to find information about my condition. The medical information that I found was nothing new; it explained airways and bowel movements, etcetera, etcetera. Boring! The medical fact that was not so boring was the average life expectancy: 18 years old.

But back to the parking lot with Katrina: that was the first time I told someone how I was really feeling. I was asking questions like: What was the point in taking anything seriously? Why should I make long-term plans? What woman would want to be involved with me? Where was God in all this? Why take loads of medicine if I'm only going to live one or two more years? That's pretty grim stuff for a 16-year-old kid to worry about. After all, many 40-year-old adults, who are supposed to be more mature and better equipped emotionally, inwardly panic at the mere thought that they are halfway through life.

As I rambled on to Katrina, pouring out all my worries and frustrations, she listened and tried to understand. She was a great listener and I am thankful she was there. What a special thing to have her company at that moment; I couldn't really unload on my parents, brothers or guy friends. I thought my parents would just dismiss me and say it was going to be all right. I thought my guy friends would have felt awkward and tossed me a beer so we could move on. I thought my brothers would tell me to suck it up. I sure as hell wasn't going to talk to a teacher or other adult and bare my soul to them. Poor Katrina—I can't remember if she said anything in particular in response, but I unloaded some heavy stuff on her and she was gracious and supportive.

Looking back, Katrina's friendship should have given me a giant insight into the nature of women. At the time I was pretty clueless about the opposite sex. Inwardly, I was also upset that I was forced to face this kind of stuff as a teenager. I thought this was the time of life when I should be focusing on things like girls, sports, and being a goofball. The worst challenge in a teen's life should be doing well in school. Off and on, I was upset that what I had to focus on was coughing in public, taking thousands of pills, getting to the bathroom before diarrhea kicked in, going to the doctor all the time, going to the hospital every summer, and being "compliant" with the multitude of treatments and therapies I was subjected to. What my shortened life expectancy *did* do was creep into my subconscious. Every time I had a major decision to make, there it was; 18 years old. Follow the logic of a teenager: why try hard in high school if I won't live long enough to go to college? Why go to college and work so hard at grades, if I won't live long enough to have a career? Why work hard at my career if I'm just going to die before achieving anything? Why take all this medicine when I'm just going to die anyway? It was difficult to see life as a long-term venture.

Short-term thinking isn't as "romantic" as you might imagine. Sure, it sounds fun to do all those things you've always wanted to do. Take risks. Go wild! Live it up! Who cares, there's no tomorrow. Sounds great, doesn't it? In reality, what short-term thinking leads to is a lot of selfish decisions. This kind of thinking typically makes you feel like you can do whatever you want because there are no consequences. When you feel that your actions have no consequences, it almost always leads you to behavior you later regret. You might have fun doing it, but you will hurt yourself and those around you. Only years later would I discover that living for *tomorrow* and beyond would be the more constructive and fulfilling path. In other words, living with *purpose*. Living for tomorrow gives us something to look forward to, instead of running away from reality (which we are really doing when we "live like there is no tomorrow").

I must admit—living like there was no tomorrow allowed me to constantly enjoy myself, and occasionally it even led to constructive activity, like climbing 14,000-foot mountains in Colorado and building a successful career. I was a "fun" guy, but I became selfish. How do you become selfish? You become reckless with the feelings of others when you don't think there is a tomorrow. To me, the feelings of my family and friends were not as important as "experiencing" life to the fullest. This way of thinking also led me to grow lax with the medicine and therapies I should have been utilizing. I *was* affected by my lack of "compliance," and if we are being honest, I am lucky to simply have survived those years. Nowadays, I often wonder: if I had focused on my life as a long-term project and taken appropriate care of myself, would my body be in better shape now? That, my friends, is what you call *regret*, and it isn't fun having that word hanging around.

For the next 15 years, I let this mid-life crisis mentality take hold in my life. What is most interesting (and quite frankly makes me feel silly, looking back) is that I was absolutely healthy. Yes, I took loads of medicine and my life expectancy was grim, but my lung functions and weight were perfect. No exaggeration—perfect! I was essentially envisioning obstacles and worst-case scenarios. I later realized that adhering to a "worst-case scenario mentality" is pointless, because life (with or without a disease) is going to throw you many challenges.

There is much good about experiencing a mid-life crisis and knowing what to do with it. It has motivated me to push my abilities and willpower and to accomplish tasks without hesitation. Notice that I didn't say "without careful thought." There is no point in waiting to do something you have passion for; if you feel a calling toward a charity… do it now! If you feel a nudge to help a stranger… dive in! If you haven't prayed in years… talk soon! Be there for somebody else… now. Plan the dream vacation. Research the new job. Envision the best possible future and you will have finished the first step in making it. Now that middle age is actually upon me… there is no crisis to be had!

Of all the people I could have told, Katrina was the best one. We remained good friends throughout high school, always sharing a special bond. I didn't perceive that our relationship could be more than friends. She happened to be in the perfect place at the perfect time, and she was the perfect person as far as I'm concerned. She certainly got more than she bargained for!

Although I did not confide in my parents during that time in my life, if it were not for their strong parental presence telling me I WAS going to college, I WILL take that medicine and I WOULD do well, I probably would not be alive today. Without my mother and father's positive outlook, I would not have achieved any of the wonderful things I have. My parents were strong enough to not allow me to fall into self-pity. They would not allow me to make decisions based on my perception of there being no tomorrow. We didn't talk about these things. They didn't seek counseling. They didn't encourage me to deal with it in a specific way. I don't know if their method was the "right way," but all I know is that I ended up accomplishing what every normal person does, and even went above and beyond that; so my parents certainly did something right.

What I now know is that, even with all the support in the world, nobody can force you to do something; nor can they make you feel better about your situation—unless you're ready to hear it. Thinking of life with a shortened life expectancy was the driving force behind all my major decisions.

Chapter 7

A FOUR-STAR LIFE

"If opportunity doesn't knock, build a door."

Milton Berle, American comedian

Brief life expectancy or not, I was an adult and doing quite well health-wise. College was finished and I was in a career that I was excelling at; but it was also a career in which I was not seeing a long-term future for me. Besides, I had an itch to "see the world" before it was too late. While I didn't necessarily have a desire to travel to exotic locales, I did desire to move away from St. Louis and live in Colorado. Remember that trip my brother Tom and I took? I had never forgotten the beautiful sights I had seen, and since that trip I wanted more than anything to move to the ski slopes, hiking trails, and always-fresh adventures of Denver.

Soon after relocating, I met a group of people who were in the upscale hotel business. Seeing a good fit, I made the hospitality business my new career. It wasn't long before I began to love my newfound work environment: lots of young people for co-workers (check). Lots of young people for clients (check). Lots of entertaining (check). Lots of traveling (check). Celebrity guests (check). Good pay (check). Free stuff (check).

Transfers to new cities every year or so. (triple check!)

Like many people starting work in a completely new field, I had to begin at the bottom and prove my worth. In order to break into the hotel business, I took a job as an administrative assistant to the sales and catering offices of an upscale hotel in a corporate area of Denver. It was an ideal position to break into the hospitality business, as the executive staff had all worked at a 5-star hotel in Denver that was owned by the same company. The team running the operation was made up of true *hoteliers* with service as their top priority. They were great mentors for anyone who had 5-star goals in their future. I had already been an assistant once and had been promoted beyond that position and given a great deal of responsibilities. For me, to take a "step back" in responsibility and level of pay was difficult. Instead of passing on the opportunity and waiting for what I thought I deserved, I took the entry-level job and was determined to prove myself so invaluable that they had to promote me. I wanted to be a manager in six months, and I made that clear to my new boss, Cara. She liked that desire, and while she couldn't promise anything, I knew she would look after me if I looked after her. Cara gave me my first "break" in this new career. She looked past my inexperience in the hotel business and saw that I strove to achieve more. I respected her position as director of sales in a well-run and demanding organization.

For my first five months, I worked hard to update the office. I accomplished more in the normal workday than previous assistants had. I learned from the sales people and listened to their advice. When the managers were out of the office, I took the initiative to help out in areas not yet in my responsibility. There were also more good people in that office than I could have hoped for. It's no coincidence that Cara hired them directly or had a large say in their hiring. In my fifth month of employment, I learned that one of my managers was moving on. My chance! I was surprised that Cara didn't immediately approach me with the job. I figured that I had worked very hard and that I had proved myself. A week went by, and a co-worker advised that I'd better go tell Cara that I wanted the job; otherwise she'd give it to someone else. I immediately got up from my desk and knocked on her door. We talked for a few minutes; turns out she had been waiting for me to take the initiative and approach her. I got the promotion.

Cara turned out to be a great boss. She helped me understand the business and she was encouraging when I was frustrated. She went to bat for me when the operations guys were griping. There was more to Cara than just being a great boss. I was often invited to have dinner with her family and go on hikes with them. Her husband, Bob, was a really easy-going guy and they were easy to spend time and relax with. A boss can easily detach herself from an employee who has challenges, but I experienced just the opposite. I was treated to someone who cared for me both as an employee and friend. It was just what I needed at that time in my life. Everyone in the office knew that I was in Denver with no family, and they made sure I was in good company on holidays and made sure I was doing well.

My Denver experience came to an abrupt end when our company was bought out by another. With less than a year under my belt in the industry, and half that much time as a manager, I had to hang on. I could tell so many stories about the new corporation and their management, but the truth is ugly and so was the character of the new leadership. That made me all the more thankful for Cara—but she was gone.

I was stuck. I had only been a manager for a couple months and still needed to prove that I could do the job well. Over the next year I worked under truly unsavory people, but I had to keep quiet and get through. I was fortunate that the other sales manager was a close friend; we plowed through the mess together. We blew away their expectations, and each time our boss would try something to undermine our efforts, we had the results to lock it down. Having completed a full year as a manager, it was acceptable in that industry to move on. I was just starting to look at other hotels when another break came with a phone call from a job recruiter: "We see you are a sales manager in Denver; would you like to interview for a job in Colorado Springs? It would most likely be more money and the hotel is a four-star establishment." I didn't hesitate for a second before saying yes to an interview.

I had a great feeling about this new opportunity. Over the phone, I could sense that my potential new boss "got" me and that I "got" him. I could hardly contain myself for the next 4 days until the interview. I'm not much of a "good omen" guy, but when the sky lit up like a Christmas tree from a shooting star overhead, I knew my interview would go well. When the entire sky behind Pikes Peak flashed bright as day several times as a meteor broke through the atmosphere, I couldn't help but feel an intense gratefulness for this new chapter I felt to be beginning.

Onward and Upward

That meteor *must* have been a good omen, because I got the job. I was again on a mission to prove I was great at my job. Perhaps more importantly, I was also out to forget about my health condition and prove that it could not hold me back. I purposefully chose a career that would give me the opportunity to move around the country (on the company's tab). I definitely wanted to experience new things and new places before it was too late. While there's nothing wrong with forming career goals, my own motivation was not from a good place. That "life expectancy thing" was still driving my decisions. At the age of 26, my life expectancy was 28—so in order for me to experience life, I reasoned, I had better get moving.

I loved my new position. The hotel in Colorado Springs was beautiful and was a perfect stepping-stone for my career. Once again, the person who hired me was on the ball. It was nice to be working in a team atmosphere after my previous year of "every man for himself." After a short time, I became one of the top sales people in the company. After a year, I was once again looking for the next opportunity. I wanted to be promoted to a position in a beautiful resort hotel on a golf course, in the mountains, or at the beach. I was eyeing several properties within my company when my management suddenly announced that our hotel was being bought out. Again! As before, the replacement for my boss was just not the same. Unfortunately for the new guy, I had already been through a less-than-excellent boss and was in no mood to return to the daily drama that poor management brings.

After the merger, my former boss moved to another company. He and I had "clicked" so well that I was hoping to work for him again. I took the initiative to call him up—by then, he had moved to the East Coast. During our conversation I let him know how I felt: neither the new company coming in nor the existing company was going to hold the right opportunity for me. I also wanted to continue my "tutelage" with him. He had been waiting for my call and he let me know that there would be something available shortly. I was excited because his new company had a complete portfolio of upscale hotels across the country. Within a couple months, I was packing my bags to move to Richmond, Virginia. I was moving to the East Coast: within shouting distance of Washington D.C., Baltimore, Philly, and the ocean! I would miss the mountains of Colorado, but this opportunity couldn't be passed up.

Spoiled

I was working in the upscale hotel business, and when you are tagged as one of those guys who can fix broken relationships with customers, you get to go to new places quite often. You also get paid well to travel. The company actually hires someone to come to your house, pack your stuff, load your stuff in a truck, and unpack it when you find a new home in a new city. In the new city, you get to stay in a beautiful hotel and receive all the goodies that go along with being a guest in an upscale hotel: room service, dry cleaning, valet parking, meals, and a $200-or-more room per night were all paid for. Although I did not get the resort job, I was with a boss that I respected greatly—and the hotel was gorgeous. It was an excellent time in my life. I was under 30 years old. I was moving around the country. I was making good money. I was somehow popular with the ladies and enjoying life very much.

The Client That Changed It All

The job in Richmond, although an excellent opportunity, was a real challenge. For 12 years, the previous sales person had not made the goal for my market segment. I knew it was going to be challenging, and that is the reason I took the job. The major blame was put on a large bank in town and one particular Vice President who was in charge of a massive amount of travel expenditures. As the person in charge of choosing a hotel to house all their employee travelers, she held a great deal of interest for my revenue goals. I heard all the horror stories about this particular lady and the difficulties others had experienced in working with her. Picky. Demanding. Hard-nosed. Impossible to make happy. (I even heard the word "witch" mentioned!) I was assured that she would never agree to a meeting with me. To me, she sounded like an ideal client for a four-star hotel; besides, I thought, aren't all successful people particular, place high expectations on those around them, and attempt to make the best deal possible? To my surprise, she was very open to a meeting with me. I knew I hadn't thrown a Jedi mind trick on her, so I figured she had something she wanted to tell me. You know, the usual speech: "Tell me a thing or two about your hotel."

She did have a thing or two to tell me. Unfortunately, she was 100% correct in her assessment of the hotel; she was extremely disappointed in us. The message brought mixed emotions. The good news was that we were messing up simple things. The bad news was that we had been messing up simple things—and that nobody had fixed them. The problem at hand was so simple that I thought I was missing something. When I approached my boss and then my boss's boss, they thought it was simple too. I told the "big boss" that if we got this particular issue fixed, we stood to gain over 10,000 "room nights" per year. This was just counting this lady's department in a large multistate bank. Even if you don't know anything about hotels, you can quickly figure her importance among our clientele.

Teaming up with the operations people, we figured out how to handle our little problem. It was such a minor detail and needed only a little bit of attentiveness and effort, but the payoff for such a small detail was huge. Within a year, we had secured all those room nights in a massive contract. Our formerly difficult client became a quiet fan of ours within her company. "Witch" or not—all she wanted was her people to be taken care of.

After a year of cleaning up Richmond, after the previous year cleaning up Colorado Springs (and the previous year exceeding expectations in Denver), I was promoted to Director of Sales. I had accomplished this goal a full year before my plan. I was the youngest Director Of Sales this company had ever promoted. My new hotel was at a beautiful upscale property. Many resources had been poured into renovations, but my company was still struggling to maintain its high-class reputation. Thinking I had the cat by the tail, I jumped at the opportunity to "turn things around." This time I wasn't just a helper—I was the guy in charge.

We had some very serious challenges with staff, operations and clientele but our new management, myself included, threw ourselves into the work. Little by little, we were changing the culture of the property and making it financially sound. Dedicating myself to a single mission started coming at a price, however. With the generous salary came a great deal of responsibility and a ton of working hours. I was so focused on achieving success and trying to forget about my health that I in fact *did* forget about my health. I forgot until I was reminded by my body—and an opportunity to speak at a charity event.

Beyond Expectations

Just before I was to move from Richmond to Detroit as part of my big promotion, I was approached by a man who had a child with the same medical condition I had. He had heard through my doctor's office that there was a guy in town who was living well with the disease his son had. He was excited to learn that I was in fact doing well and had given a few motivational speeches in the past. The man explained that there was to be a large black tie fundraiser, and the organizers wanted *me* to be the keynote speaker. Before I agreed to do it, however, I had to do some homework on all things related to my disease. Until that point, I had been very much out of touch with the medical community and research relating to my condition. What were the new medicines? What were the new therapies? What was happening with fund-raising? What was the current life expectancy?

In my preparation for the speech, I got a pretty big shock. I found out that the life expectancy for me was 28. I had just turned 30. This was the first time in my life I was BEYOND my life expectancy. Since my sixteenth birthday, I had been making major decisions based on the knowledge that my life was going to be cut short. I had always been looking down the end of a gun barrel, but that way of thinking and those self-defenses I put up were going to have to change. My "life view" was going to start changing in big ways. For the short term, though, I had a speech to give, a big new job to prepare for, and a move.

At the black tie gala, many families whose children had my disease approached me. They were in such awe of me. Now, I enjoy attention and I like recognition. Admittedly, I'm a sort of recognition addict—but this was different. I wasn't sure that I liked *this* at all. What had I done to deserve such admiration? I was just a young guy working hard and experiencing career success. Honesty, I really hadn't achieved anything many other young achievers hadn't. It felt very strange when people told me things like: you're 30 years old. You have a career, live an active lifestyle—and you're alive. What a weird thing, to be admired because you're 30 years old and like to do stuff other 30-year-old guys like to do. These are such simple, normal things.

The very next day after the gala, I said my farewells in Virginia and made the trek to Michigan. I had little time to ponder the opportunities that this unique life was delivering. Upon settling in at my new hotel, the work was fast and furious. The problems at this property were numerous. The building was still a problem after millions of dollars of renovation. As the Director of Sales, it was difficult for me to see employees who took no pride in their work. The fact that our customers were also unhappy was a huge setback for our revenue. I decided that if all went well, I could fix my part of the problem and be rewarded within a couple years with a position at a beautiful new hotel property with no problems. That was the path I planned on.

I stayed focused, but very soon I felt the effects of working too many hours and not exercising or taking the treatments my body so badly needed. Soon I was sick. I remembered the last time I worked too hard and the series of events that followed. Work too many hours. No exercise. No treatments. No appetite. Lose 10 pounds. Lose 10% lung capacity. Lose relationships with the ones I love. Risk death.

The pattern was repeating, and I knew at that moment that I had big decisions to make. Was I going to continue to ignore my body and achieve career success until it wiped me out? Or was I going to focus on taking care of my body so I could have a chance at living a few more years? Was I going to move back to Colorado? What new career could I take up, one that didn't require so many hours? What lifestyle choices would I have to make that were better suited to a chronic condition?

These were only secondary questions, though. The big question was this: how long was I going to let this disease dictate how I thought of my life?

Chapter 8

CHASING YOUR TAIL

"Hope emerges in the shattering experience of living despite all hope."

Johann Baptist Metz, German theologian

I had made my decision, and that decision was to take charge of my physical health. My decision came with an important promise: I was not going to let this disease negatively dictate the way I thought ever again. As I began to think more about this decision and the changes it would bring about, there was an image that would not leave my mind: a picture of a dog chasing its tail. You've seen it. Poor little animal going around and around and eventually exhausting itself. The interesting thing to me—and the reason this image is ingrained in my mind—is that the dog never catches its tail. (Not that I've seen, anyway.) Doesn't tail-chasing seem like a colossal waste of energy on the dog's part? When I had finally outlived my life expectancy, I figured I had wasted a lot of energy and years chasing the ghost of death. Throughout my youth, the ghost was always just in front of me yet out of reach; and now I had grabbed the ghost—but I was very much alive. I'm glad that I

61

have moved on from thoughts that were so limiting.

In order to take charge of my health and be closer to the people I knew would help if I needed it, I made the decision to move back home. I admitted that my health could change on a moment's notice and that I might require having loved ones around. Being practical for the first time in a long time, I moved back home with a new attitude and a new mission.

After arriving in St. Charles, I felt unsettled with my job. I felt unsettled with my social life. I felt unsettled about living in the Midwest. I felt unsettled about what to do about changing my life and becoming somebody different. Moving back home was the most unsettling thing I had ever done. I felt as if I had to start again at "square one," and I had no idea how best to proceed. I had moved from St. Louis to Denver, from Denver to Colorado Springs, from Colorado Springs to Richmond, from Richmond to Detroit, Michigan—all in the span of five years. Within those five years, I had survived two mergers and an assortment of new bosses, and had lived in eight different homes. With each move I had to adjust to new personalities at work, form new relationships with clients, and somehow make new friends.

Yet moving home and "settling in" caused the most anxiety of all.

Looking back, the factor that was greatly contributing to my anxiety was how to live with this chronic illness. I had no answers, but I was determined to stick to this new resolution of taking better care of myself. I wouldn't push it aside, so I might as well go at it straight ahead. I was tired of being fearful and trying to ignore something that couldn't be ignored. No matter what I did, "it" was always there and constantly stalking me.

My new pervasive thoughts were less about worry and more about the realization that I only had control over one thing in my life. I realized that I only had influence on my physical body. The disease I have will sometimes just do what it does regardless of the medicine and therapies I do. The weather is not in my control. My bosses are not in my control; nor are my clients, parents, brothers, or friends. The one thing I have complete control of is the thought in my mind at any one time. Oh yes, people are often competing for ownership of that thought, but I remain in control of it. My own life experiences and current circumstances were tugging for influence over my thoughts, but I was learning to take back ownership.

I learned to listen to my thoughts. I often caught myself in a spiral of "what if's" going on inside my head. Many times, whether it was thoughts of life with this disease, work, or relationships, I would start with imagining made-up scenarios in my head. This imagining can sometimes be constructive. We see professional athletes envisioning success before their race. Golfers, I think, are most famous for this, as they "see" where the ball is going before swinging. In the oft-quoted movie *Caddyshack*, Chevy Chase tells his young protégé: "Be the ball, Danny." More times than I'd like to admit, my own internal dialogue would tend to the negative. When I learned to actually hear those thoughts and recognize when I was turning negative, things started to change. Stopping the negative "what if's" was a big step in training my brain to find a positive approach. Reversing those thoughts would prove key in truly moving forward, and would be critical in completely overcoming my challenges.

At this time, I had a co-worker who was a recovering alcoholic. He had struggled with his addiction for years. For decades he had pushed people away, and although he had gone through rehab, he was not embracing an attitude of change. So nothing changed— until he made the decision to get his life back together. I asked him what made the difference this time and why he had chosen to better himself after all those years. He responded by letting me know that he *wanted* to change. Well, there you have it. All those years of struggle could have been washed away if he simply *wanted* it. I'm not telling you that it was easy for him once he embraced the desire to overcome his addiction. I'm simply stating that until he made this decision, everything good and constructive bounced off him like that fortress wall I mentioned earlier in this book. This was not the only factor in his life's change, but his conscious

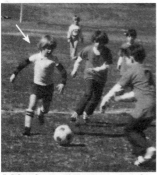

decision is what it boiled down to. I truly connected with him on this point, and it reinforced my growing notion that the life you want is simply one decision away... followed by a whole lot of work.

A History of "Staying Active"

As a child, my parents were told by my doctors to "keep Michael active," so I played a lot of team sports. By high school,

Mike playing soccer in 1st grade

I was not fast enough, tall enough or strong enough to play any team sport competitively. I was never ultra-competitive or a great athlete, but I liked playing games when it meant something. Many a competitive wiffle ball game was played with my buddies in those years. Growing up, there were many signs as to what I could do well.

Late in high school, my older brother Matt bought a bicycle and was riding it quite a bit. He made riding bikes sound like fun, and I looked up to my brothers, so this idea was interesting. The person that most convinced me to try cycling was Greg LeMond, a famous cyclist who won the Tour de France in 1986, 1989 and 1990. He was the first American to win that prestigious race. In 1989, when he was close to possibly repeating his title, the national news was filled with stories of his attempt. In 1989 he battled the famous Frenchman Laurent Fignon, a two-time champion of the Tour de France making a comeback of his own. Their three-week epic battle in 1989 ended up being the closest Tour de France margin of victory, with LeMond's winning by a mere 8 seconds. What struck me most was that LeMond was battling injuries from a horrific earlier accident, in which he nearly died. After two years of rehabilitation he was competing in the most difficult race a cyclist can attempt. His story of overcoming challenge appealed to me greatly. I was particularly drawn to this sport because of the ability of these men to ride for hours every day for three weeks straight. Their speeds were incredibly fast, averaging over 20 miles an hour for hours at a time. All this speed was highlighted by a grueling week or so in the high mountains of the Alps and Pyrenees. My mind was enthralled at the fitness level required to cycle up mountains for hours at a time. It was also very exciting that they would reach speeds of 60+ mph on the way down those mountains.

The Cycling Adventure

Wrapped in the awe of Greg LeMond and the Tour de France, I bought a bike. I discovered an obsession of sorts with endurance. I absolutely loved being on the road for hours without anybody around. Riding in the countryside with no cars or people around was bliss. With only the smooth hiss of bicycle tires on the road and the wind in my ears, I could zone out and immerse myself in my thoughts.

On one such ride between the cornfields near the Mississippi

River, I was somewhere other than St. Charles County in my mind. In the middle of my reverie, I was rudely shaken from my interior world by a madly barking dog. He came blazing out from behind a farmhouse, barking as if I were a grizzly bear attacking his master. When his barking snapped me out of my beautiful mental zone, I noticed he was coming *really* fast. I was already doing nearly 20 mph, but he obviously had the sprinting ability to match that. It was fun racing him for a second, until I truly realized I was going to be his meal. Just before nipping my heels, he received a squirt from my water bottle. As he broke off his chase in a clumsy, snorting stumble, I laughed that uncomfortable laugh that comes when you realize things could have gone worse. I would have to remember this farmhouse and be prepared to practice sprinting in the future. That crazed dog also made me realize that in my "zone" I had pedaled many miles without feeling or thinking about the effort. I understood what the "zone" was now and how endurance athletes can comfortably exercise for so long. Other than the occasional dog, I found this type of riding soothing. Soon 50 miles on the bicycle became routine.

A friend knew of my riding and a co-worker of his was an avid cyclist. The co-worker wanted to ride in the Multiple Sclerosis 150 (MS 150), which is a two-day, 150-mile bike ride. This ride would take us nearly halfway across Missouri, and on the first day we would tackle the dreaded "7 Hills Of Herman." I didn't know what they were, but the bikers I knew were dreading those seven hills. It didn't help that those hills would come *after* 60 miles of biking.

This was right up my alley. I immediately signed up for the ride.

Training for and completing the MS 150 provided a fun way for me to exercise and stay active and focused. My doctors were very pleased because my lung functions were above 100% at the time. Although bicycling served me well in those years, bicycling requires an inordinate amount of time, so I couldn't regularly cycle to battle this disease. With the experience of the MS 150 in my mind, I knew something special could be done even in spite of my disease, and that I was capable of a great deal of athletic activity.

During my college years, I also ran quite a bit when I didn't have much time for other athletics. I was a good runner, but I didn't *love* it. Even though it wasn't a passion, it was the exercise option that made sense for time commitment and my doctors liked it best. I coughed a lot more during running than biking and that meant airway clearance. Now, all those years later and back at home in St. Charles, I began to run again. I ran a couple miles at a time, a few days a week. Running like this soon became tedious, however. When the weather wasn't perfect I didn't run; when the weather was downright nasty, I didn't even pretend I wanted to run. Without the goal of making a soccer team or getting in shape for some particular event, running was useless. Who runs just to run? I knew of a couple people who ran just for the sport of it and they were in great shape, but I continually asked myself how I could keep running interesting and keep myself motivated.

What's So Hard About Running...

Making things more difficult was the shape my lungs were in at this stage. I really didn't know how much my disease had progressed until I started running. A few years of little exercise and little therapy had taken its toll. Each time I would rededicate myself to running again, the first days out were miserable with coughing. It's very frustrating to try to find a rhythm when you cough so hard you throw up. While that gave me a perfect excuse to buy cool new shoes, it was devastating to motivation. I found out it wasn't only the first couple of days this would happen. Anytime I worked up a significant amount of mucus from deep within my lungs, it had the chance of getting stuck. It would usually get stuck right in that spot in your throat that makes you gag. Each time I attempted to run further or faster, I would loosen up more crap in my lungs that would trigger a coughing fit.

On top of the coughing, I hadn't figured out what to eat so I wouldn't have diarrhea. I had to figure out how to get my digestion under control so I didn't have to run so close to a bathroom. Not only did I have to figure out how to avoid stomach issues, but I had to figure out how to eat right. What foods caused indigestion? What foods were easy to digest? What foods were nutritionally optimal for runners, especially runners who don't digest food very well? How would I fit in eating right with a 40-hour-a-week job? Between the shape of my lungs and trying to figure out how to get my stomach right, my work was cut out for me. With the help of doctors, running peers, and lots of experimenting, I was figuring these things out. I just hadn't figured out yet how to make things *interesting*.

In my search for making running "more than therapy," I also wanted to do something not everyone would attempt. I wanted to do something everyone *could* do and at the same time do something not everyone would *want* to do. I knew loads and loads of people who ran 5K/3.1 mile races. I'd even run a couple of those as a kid. I'd already run a 10K/6.2 mile race, and there were 50,000 other people running that race. Nothing special with those distances; been there, done that. What was far enough to set this goal far apart from anything I'd tried before? What was that goal that would prove I was doing something not everyone would want or dare to try and do?

Total Inspiration

What about a *marathon*? Could I do 26.2 miles of non-stop running, as fast as possible? That seemed a terribly long distance, and besides, how could that be done with my condition? This idea had been simmering in my mind for years and was now coming to a boil. At that time, I had two friends training for a marathon, my college roommate and my sister-in-law, who were both knee-deep into training. I was encouraged by the fact that they were seemingly average athletes with no grand athletic prowess or running background. Keeping in contact with them and hearing how they were methodically attempting this goal fanned the flames of my courage. As they ran into double-digit mileage, I was not only curious, but also impressed by their dedication. They really had to dedicate themselves to training—but the kicker is that they were talking like it was fun. It reminded me of hearing about cycling for the first time, when my brother said *that* was fun.

My curiosity was at its peak and I wanted to get a better sense of what a marathon was like. I went up to Chicago with a buddy to watch my sister-in-law (technically she is my sister-in-law's sister, but for brevity's sake I'll refer to her as an in-law) run her first marathon. On race day, we rushed from spot to spot to see her. From the start line we hustled over to Mile 3. From Mile 3 we hurried over to Mile 13.1. From 13.1 we hastily got back to the finish line. The entire time we were in the midst of thousands upon thousands of spectators chasing runners hoping to catch a fleeting glimpse of their own superstar. Of all the spots we watched runners, my favorite spot was Mile 13.1. Halfway point. The runners come down a big four-lane boulevard into a downtown district. As they approached the halfway mark, high-rise buildings created a stadium-like effect, where noise bounced from one side of the street to the other, making the spectators' cheering sound like half-crazed college students at a National Championship game. Right at the halfway mark, the runners took a sharp right turn and the stadium effect was multiplied by thousands of people camped on the rising steps that led up to an office building. Spectators were equipped with whatever objects made the most noise. Clanging cowbells, shrieking whistles, boom boxes set on tables, drums, and of course their own frantic yelling. One guy was seemingly just cheering for anybody who ran by. "Hey Number 412—you got great legs!"

This was *fun*.

The first individuals to come by were in wheelchairs. I didn't know wheelchair athletes existed at the marathon distance. Amazing! They were going incredibly fast and powered only by the strength of their arms. (Nice guns, I thought.) The next individuals to come by were the elite runners. Just a couple of men trickling by, and they were in an all-out sprint. I was calculating their speed and had to ask my buddy if my math was correct. It was indeed correct and it blew me away that they could run that fast for so long. One after the other, with short gaps between them, the leaders were screaming by and not looking one bit like they had already run 13.1 miles. Gazelles had been let loose in the streets of Chicago, I mused. Next through came the female leaders. They were running faster than I could imagine. Smooth and effortless. Imagining that I could do this was intimidating but exciting at the same time. The elite runners looked all the same. Both men and women were lean, had long legs, and their age was somewhere between 25 to 35 years old. After the leaders went shooting by, there was a lull. Finally, a few more runners appeared. The professionals had gone by and now there was a mix of guys and girls, and each looked amazingly fluid and strong. A few minutes later, the pack had grown thicker and I was having a hard time picking out any single runner. In a few minutes the four-lane boulevard was absolutely packed from curb to curb with a sea of runners. They were not going as fast as the leaders, but they were still cruising along. Now the runners looked tall and short, skinny and not so skinny, old and young—a huge mix of physiques. I even saw "Captain America" run by. Somebody was doing this for absolute fun. The crowd had grown since we first got there and was now whipped up and feeding off each other. The runners were yelling back at the crowd and exchanging high fives. I felt exhilarated; the energy was palpable.

Missing my sister-in-law among the tens of thousands of runners, we hustled back to the finish line to catch her there. I wasn't expecting a long stretch of bleachers and countless throngs of people to be at the finish. All these people were at a marathon? This wasn't the Olympics or anything—I was amazed at the sheer size of the crowd that had come to witness a seemingly average running event. Hoping to see her at the finish, we got a spot on the bleachers within sight of the finish line. We could see the runners making the final sprint down a long straight stretch. It was a perfect spot. As the runners were going by, there was a range of emotions. Some were shouting to the crowd with arms raised in anonymous victory. Others saw a family member and came toward the bleachers to blow a kiss or give a thumbs-up. All had the finish line in their sights and were pouring on the gas. I was amazed that some of these runners had enough energy to jump over the finish line or turn a handspring after 26 miles of running. You could see the prize in the runners' eyes and feel the excitement of the crowd. When a runner would pass and their friends would see them, a hail of shouting would go out for that runner. "Go Mom!" "You did it Dad!" "I love you, you've done it!"

All this was terribly exciting and was capped off with the best sight I'd seen in my life. A middle-aged man was running hard, looking like he was going to finish well. Then suddenly he pulled up and started hopping. He had cramped up and it must have hurt something fierce to stop just meters away from the finish. He was in so much discomfort that he hobbled over to the barricades in front of the bleachers. His legs were locked up and he looked like Frankenstein, walking stiffly. The grimace on his face and grunts of pain said it all. The crowd was going absolutely nuts yelling for him. They were shouting encouragement and urging him to get going, as the finish line was just meters away. When he gained the strength to continue and turned toward the finish, the crowd roused up another round of cheers and he pumped his fist to show us we were heard. It was a fist pump full of exhaustion, but we got the message loud and clear.

We witnesses were thinking we'd seen it all when we spotted a young woman. She was running her heart out down the stretch, clearly racing another runner, as they were side-by-side for a long time. She was looking great! Like the gentleman before her, all of a sudden she stumbled to a stop. She was a sweaty mess, bending over with her hands on her knees. Gathering some last energy, she took a few steps to get out of the way of approaching runners. She shuffled toward the side of the road where thousands of onlookers watched. The crowd was wondering aloud what she was experiencing. All eyes were fixed on her. With her hands on her knees, facing the crowd, her body suddenly tightened into a wracking convulsion and with a giant wretch, she threw up violently. It seemed as though a gallon of water was coming out of her body, which was in full revolt. She was shaking from exhaustion. When she let it out, the crowd gave a collective gasp. Before she could collect herself, the crowd was frantically cheering her to get going. I was yelling "Go! Go! Go!" along with the screaming crowd. With a miraculous bit of energy, she sprinted to the end. In the next hour there were numerous runners who had given it their entire being to finish. Some vomited, some had to stop and stretch out, and others had to walk it in. Whenever somebody stopped, the gigantic crowd would start yelling at them to finish, finish, finish.

Seeing the runners give their all was fascinating. It reminded me of the 1984 Olympics in Los Angeles. Gabriela Andersen-Schiess was in the inaugural field of the Women's Olympic Marathon. On television I watched her stagger across the finish line, and it was awe-inspiring to my 14-year-old self. Her story is all the more inspiring to me now, as I know women were almost not allowed to participate in the 1984 Olympic Marathon. By God, she would finish the race, if for no other reason than she committed to it. Watching those average marathon runners who would never win a race give all of themselves to a goal made complete sense to me as a 30-year-old. THAT was what I wanted to do. Not stagger across the finish line, mind you, but push the limits of what I thought I could do. To truly challenge my body and mind, and in the meantime, to kick my disease right where it hurt.

My mind was set on 26.2 miles!

Obsession

How would my body and this disease factor in? Let me tell you first about the three things runners obsess about. One is a little thing called VO2Max. Two is nutrition. Three is hydration.

V02Max is a measure of the body's ability to process oxygen. Without getting extremely technical, mostly because I can't, VO2Max specifically indicates one's capacity for aerobic endurance. The truly great runners and cyclists have V02Max numbers off the chart. Starting with the 80% lung capacity of a normal 30-year-old, I was looking at a serious handicap even before starting.

Nutrition is also of utmost importance. Most runners I know change their eating habits regularly to enhance their performance. To oversimplify the issue, you can't run very fast or very long with White Castle as your fuel. A runner's diet has specific nutritional requirements, especially as you stack on marathon training mileage. Runners watch carbohydrate and protein intake and shoot for specific ratios of carbs to protein. What they eat on Monday through Thursday is different than what they eat on Friday and Saturday. What they eat before a run is different than what they eat after a run. Running magazines spend endless articles on sports nutrition. This is not even mentioning the countless options for nutritional supplements. Here I was, having to already take over 10,000 pills a year simply to digest food. Even with those pills, my body processes a fraction of the nutritional value of the food I eat.

Hydration is the final obsession for runners. It is said that a 3% dehydration rate in the body produces a 15% reduction in performance. In short, make darn sure you drink plenty of fluid and the *right* kind of fluid at the *right* rate of intake. Again, there is a science to this, and if you're going to perform optimally you better get it right. Too much fluid and you can die of hyponatremia. Too little fluid and you can die of heat stroke—or at a minimum cramp up so badly you can't finish. This body of mine does not regulate chloride on a cellular level. This is why mucus in my body gets so thick and plugs up airways and digestive enzyme secretions. What it also does is create an inordinate amount of salt loss in sweat. Salt is filled with electrolytes, which regulate our hydration and are critical for nerve and muscle function. As a result of the extra salt in my sweat, I lose an abnormally high amount of electrolytes when exercising. There is a whole industry surrounding electrolyte replenishment, with the most famous company being Gatorade. Logically, you can assume the following formula would be accurate:

Reduced Lung Capacity + *Bad Digestion* + *Excessive Electrolyte Loss* = Horrible Runner Body.

Let's just say I had my work cut out for me, but I didn't care what handicaps my body was supposed to present. I was *going* to do this.

Chapter 9

RACE DAY

*"Life is either a daring adventure,
or nothing at all."*

Helen Keller, American author and activist

The Long Road For One Day

So began my own journey to 26.2 miles. I wasn't completely oblivious to the difficulty of the task, so I bought a book to teach me how to go the distance. I began to run beyond a few miles, a few days a week. I began to dedicate myself to the mileage required every day; one step in front of the other. I easily got up to 8 miles on my Saturday long run. A quick lesson in running: each day you run different distances and at different speeds to gain endurance fitness. On a weekly basis, it culminates in a "long run" on Saturday or Sunday. This long run is designed to prepare the body and the mind for hours of non-stop exercise.

Upon attempting 10 miles on my weekly long run, I was very nervous. I had just completed 8 miles with relative ease, but 10 miles was double digits. That seemed like a big deal. To be safe, I outlined the roads I would be taking and gave the route to my parents. Their instructions were that if they didn't hear from me in two hours, come to where I was running, find my limp and helpless body, and peel me off the pavement. Well, I finished the 10 miles with ease, and was brimming full of confidence. My friends and family thought I was a bit nutty. The most common question I was being asked was simply "Why?" I didn't want to go into all the reasons, so I just stole Sir Edmund Hilary's line about climbing Mt. Everest: "Because it's there." Secretly, I enjoyed the fact that people were baffled. It meant I was doing something special; so I kept pushing.

Twelve, thirteen and fourteen-mile runs came and went, and I was as strong as the first 6-mile run weeks ago. This was just too easy. I was getting very excited about the race in a couple months. It was time for 16 miles—which you would have thought would be daunting, since 10 miles seemed such a milestone. Not so. I was really full of confidence as I set off for 16 miles. 8 miles out and 8 miles back. As I was cruising along, I started feeling a bit fatigued. I hadn't felt tired on any of my previous runs… honestly. I thought it was probably just lack of water, or that I didn't stretch enough, or that this is just how serious mileage feels and that it would pass. A few minutes later I was lying on my back on the side of the road. My back muscles had clenched up, which had sent my neck into a spasm. I plopped down as fast as I could so as not to free-fall. I must have looked like a fish out of water, rolling from side to side and alternating stretching and freezing so as to not further the cramping. I'm sure I looked ridiculous. After a few frightening minutes, I was looser and able to stand up. I tried running slowly, but my body was having none of that. So I started the long walk back. It was close to 4 miles from the car, and I was walking in considerable discomfort. Leaning to one side so my back wouldn't flip out again, I trudged to the car. I was so bummed out.

Being stubborn and lacking a normal sense of caution about what I was attempting, the following Saturday I set out to accomplish 16 miles again. This was scheduled as a 13-mile day. It was supposed to be an "active recovery" run in which the miles reduce for a week, but I wanted to hit that 16 to prove something. So I made adjustments of more water intake the day before, more carbs for dinner the night before, and good stretching.

With a few miles to go I was on the ground again, back flipping out, and my neck extremely sore—mere blocks away from where I was the previous weekend. If you think I was bummed the first time, I was devastated the second. Looking ahead to race day, I only had a few weeks to go, and next week was 18 miles. If you can't run 16 you can't run 18. If you can't run 18 you sure as heck can't run 26.2. I was freaking out. My unreasonable lack of caution was gone. My confidence was shot. I had already put some 12 to 14 weeks of training into this effort; was it going to end on this note?

You Get By With A Little Help...

To quote John Wayne in the movie *Big Jake:* "Not hardly." I got smart and asked for some help. Apparently, reading a book, being stubborn, and possessing determination weren't enough to complete 26.2 miles. There was more strategy involved. I wanted to do well, and I was willing to get the help I needed. I went to my favorite running store and told the experienced runners there what was happening. They asked me a question I thought I had answered already. (I had answered it, but not correctly. It was not the first time that had happened in my life!) Their answer was so simple: they told me to drink Gatorade instead of water during my run. In addition, they told me not to eat energy bars during my run, but to eat GU Energy Gel instead. GU is a pudding-like substance you can eat during a run; it gives you instant energy while requiring minimal digestive energy from the body. Considering my intense electrolyte loss and inability to digest food, this substance seemed like a dream come true for me.

Saturday rolled around again, and 18 miles loomed large. By this time I already had two attempts at 16, so my scheduled mileage was even higher. My estimated time for 18 miles was 3 hours. For the first time in my running "career," I was overly nervous. My route was going to take me far past town, out to middle of farm fields. Past where there would be any traffic at 5:30AM. Almost to the Mississippi River AND back. The sheer time on my feat was growing more daunting in my mind.

Loaded with new knowledge, I put my worries aside and focused on my pace. Aside from checking my watch every mile and staying on top of hydration, I let my mind grow excited about what I was doing. The miles started to click off and I was doing great. Mile 1: Feeling nervous and determined at the same time. Mile 3: It was still barely light. Mile 5: Off the city streets and hitting the little county highway with 6-foot tall corn on both sides. Mississippi River in front of me and Missouri River to my back. Mile 8: Crossing the train tracks. I used to ride my bike this way in college and thought it was really far. Time to turn around.

Time for a body check. Feeling great. Legs are strong. No cramping in my back. Neck is loose. Feet are perfect. Time for a mind check. I'm still focused. I'm enjoying this! I can't believe I'm running this far. True, there is nobody around to help if I need it. But I don't need it. Feeling great.

Heading back. The sun is just peeking over the trees. It's going to start getting warm when that sun gets over those trees. How's my hydration? Plenty left. I'm not even sweating a lot. Awesome! Mile 10, 11 and 12. Click. Click. Click. 6 miles to go. Body check. Legs strong. Back and neck relaxed. Hips are tight. Just listen to your body and if it gets bad we'll take it as it comes. Doesn't hurt, but I can feel it. Mile 13: I feel awesome, with only five miles to go. I'm back in the city streets. Couple-mile stretch here and I'm as good as done. How's my time? Sweet, I'm fast. Maybe I should go faster? *Nope. Stay with the game plan.* 18 miles at a steady pace is the goal. How many people with your condition have done this? Not many. I'm awesome! I should be an Olympian...

Holy cow, my mind was wondering. I'm at 15 miles. Hey wait! I'm further than the last two weeks where I broke down. I got *that* monkey off my back. 3 miles to go. Home stretch. Body check: legs strong. Back loose. Hip doesn't hurt anymore. Don't need a mind check because I just zoned out. Those miles go fast when you're zoned out.

18 MILES... DONE! Body check. I feel great. I could go even further. Mind check: I enjoyed that challenge. Man, I am confident again. Time check. I ran the first 16 miles faster than I ran 13 previously and added two miles with that pace. Glad I got some help from the running store. Geniuses!

18 miles. I never really processed that mileage along with 3 hours when I first started to train and it was probably a good thing. If you look at 18 miles at Week 1 of training, you can easily think it is impossible. Luckily I thought more like this: I've run 6 miles already so surely I can run 8. If I can run 8 then

I can run 10. I f I could run 15, I could run 16. I looked at 26.2 miles like this.

I also look at my life like this. I have my major goal in mind: to stay healthy and be 100% compliant. If I looked at all my medicine and therapies needed over a lifetime, I would probably pass out. What I *can* do is look at my daily routine and make the necessary adjustments to my life to make that happen. Life becomes possible when taken one day at a time. My friend Kristen often reminds new runners that you can't eat an elephant at one time. We have to break up our big goals into manageable and achievable bits so we don't get overwhelmed.

Training for a marathon is an 18-week process to change the body. From the way you look in the mirror to the way your body processes energy on a cellular level, big changes occur. Activities that were difficult physically mere weeks before become easy. A mental change occurs as well: you gain confidence, determination, and discipline. You learn to make a plan and adjust if necessary. Curiously enough, things that were mentally difficult mere weeks ago are now easy. In training for my marathon, my challenges with my disease took on another personality, so to speak. My approach was something like this: Eat better so I can have a good run. Take all those pills so I can have a good run. Do the lung treatments so I can have a good run. Don't overwork so I can get in a good run. Don't drink too much so I can get in a good run. I was so focused on having *good runs* that I truly embraced all the things I previously hated making time for. For the first time in my life, I was not running away from this disease, but doing something about it. I was kicking its butt for a change.

To Toe the Line

Race day was drawing near. It was only a month or so away, and that meant only a few more weeks of hard training, then an easier week or two of what runners call "the taper," which is a period of easier running that allows the body to fully recover from months of constant work. During "the taper" one goes a bit nutty. It generally means too much free time and energy for a person who has dedicated many months to exercising long hours every day. It is a time when you look forward to the race tremendously. The hard work is done. You have broken in any new shoes or clothing. You know what you will eat and drink days before the race. Travel plans have long been made, and it's cruising time.

I was ready to taper and all was set for race day—when a longtime friend called and asked me to be in his wedding. Of course I wanted to celebrate with them, so I asked when the wedding was to take place. You guessed it, the very weekend of my race. What's the problem, you might ask? The 18 weeks of training were built around *this* particular weekend. All the accumulated miles, and then the tapering, were building to a very specific peak date. Even if, logistically speaking, I could have worked out my wedding travel, I wasn't going to break the routine. The perfect foods. The perfect amounts of food. Good sleep. Good hydration. All these things are carefully attended to leading up to the race, and, at least for me, a wedding means eating like crazy, drinking a few drinks that don't count toward hydration, and lots of cake. Not to mention a few long nights with little rest.

Bottom line is, I was going to my friends' wedding, but my relaxing taper time was done for because I had to locate another marathon. The new marathon date had to be within a week or two of the scheduled race. There are only so many 26.2-mile races in the Midwest. On top of geographic limitations, I had to hit that "peak time" I had been preparing for six months. I had a very limited window where I could reschedule without major changes to training. I started to search the Internet. Where could I get to? Would I have to find flights? Hotels? Would rescheduling this late in the game cost a fortune? The race had to be fairly close. I searched and searched and finally found a race within a day's drive of my home. I was so excited. Dad had already agreed to take his R.V. if needed, so I called to get registered for the race. Until that phone call, I had never heard of a "private" marathon; turns out that this marathon I found after so much searching was not open to the public. So frustrating! But I found a way around this—I gave the race director my "sob story" and threw in my medical condition to garner some goodwill, and he became very excited to have me come to their race. We'll get to what the *Runners Club* is later, because that group blew my mind in the end.

So I was settled and had everything back under control. I had mixed emotions because the new race weekend was conflicting with my mom's availability. She had already committed to babysitting my niece and nephew in Indianapolis that weekend. She was going to make a special trip there and my parents aren't the kind of people to back out of anything. I was disappointed, but mom was one hundred times sadder, although she was grateful we would be able to have some father and son time. In the end, Dad and I were going to have a fun weekend; it was going to be great to take a road trip with him.

I had worked hard and completed every workout with the timeliness and diligence of a Marine Corps drill sergeant. Although I had a couple of nervous weeks, not for one second did I let doubt overtake my will to finish this thing. Apparently I was the only one *not* worried. As good parents should be, my Mom and Dad had concerns about this new endeavor. They too remembered the images of Olympians collapsing on race day.

Most marathons have anywhere from a couple thousand to 50,000 runners. This race had 250. Who were these people having their own race? They actually picked Tulsa, Oklahoma? (Can I ask why, in heaven's name?) Not that Tulsa is bad, but of all the beautiful and exciting places in the United States to visit, they had picked Tulsa? I was so curious. The race director was such a pleasant guy. He invited me to the group's pasta dinner the night before the race. How nice was that? Dad and I went to the hotel where the dinner was being served and were seated with five others. By now, we knew the name of the club and had some idea as to what they were all about, but we were about to get a serious shock.

The *50 States Marathon Club*. These nuts wanted to run a marathon in every state. Fifty marathons? Who could do that? But it gets better: at my table there were two women from Chicago. These ladies were something else—they had already walked at least 10 marathons around the country, clicking off each state. Wow! Ten marathons. They were no spring chickens, either. There was more, though. There were two gentlemen sitting with me and Dad, and they told us they had run many dozens of marathons, and as a matter of fact, after they were done with the Tulsa Marathon they were showering up and getting in the car to drive to Goodland, Kansas, that same day. Why Kansas, you ask? To run a marathon on the very next day. Two marathons in two days. I trained six months for *one*. These guys were animals!

As the dinner went on, they gave talks recognizing some

of their members. Who had traveled the furthest? (London, England.) Who was the youngest? (Sixteen.) This went on and each time I was blown away. Then they came to the last two awards. The oldest, 82 years old. This guy was at my table. I thought he was there cheering on someone else. 82! I thought I had better beat the old man—I was only 31! The final award went to "Big English" Dave. Who had run the most marathons? Over 700. I could hardly believe my ears! Did I pick the worst marathon to run for the first time, or the best? I was clearly a rank amateur in the midst of marathon giants.

Even so, that night was so encouraging. Many people had heard my story and that I was decades beyond my life expectancy. They'd heard that I had trouble breathing normally and had trouble digesting food normally. The interest the club showed in my story was overwhelming. It was quite possibly the best marathon I could have entered, and it was all by accident. Most of the people looked normal. They were tall and short, fat and skinny; they were young and most certainly old. And there were others that looked like the poster child for marathoners. I liked these people immensely. They had passion for marathons and were enthusiastic to welcome a newbie like myself.

About halfway through dinner, I noticed that my dad was not in the room. I had been so enthralled with the goings-on and talking to these amazing people that I hadn't noticed he was gone. I figured he was in the bathroom or outside getting some fresh air. Or, more likely, he had gotten to chatting with someone and I just didn't see him. About halfway through dinner, he came through the doors with my brother Tom. I didn't know if anybody else from my family was going to make it, and seeing him was unbelievable. Tom had always been encouraging and was curious about my progress over the months. He had flown in from St. Louis, just to be my own personal cheerleader. The night was turning into a perfect set up for the race, which was now 12 hours away. After we said our goodnights to those amazing people, I thanked the club profusely and left feeling higher than a kite.

One doesn't sleep much the night before their first 26.2-mile race. Even before a "normal" race I would be excited, but with the people I had just met and my brother surprising me, there was no way I was sleeping, so lying awake I envisioned my run. I recalled what all those great workouts felt like. I envisioned hitting my target pace and what that would feel like. I was so thankful that I was healthy enough to even be doing it in the first place. I realized that over the previous six months, I had conquered my obsession with the negative thoughts living with a chronic disease can bring. I turned something very negative in my life to something unbelievably positive. With these thoughts in mind, I finally fell asleep.

Race morning was perfect! Cool temperatures. Overcast sky, but no rain. An enthusiastic crowd. Flat course. Family for support. (All a boy needs!) After saying hello to my tablemates from the previous night, we sang the National Anthem and the starting gun went off. I must admit, I don't remember many details mile by mile. I remember feeling good almost the entire time. I had twinges of frustration that I was being passed by so many people, but I kept reminding myself to run my race. During the famous USA vs. USSR hockey game during the 1980 Winter Olympics, coach Herb Brooks told his players to "play your game." Good advice, Herb! Ten minutes per mile wouldn't make records, but that was my goal. Calming the competitive streak in me, I focused on the fact that a ten-minute-per-mile goal would be respectable for a guy who takes over 10,000 pills a year and has limited lung capacity.

I do remember very clearly a couple things. First, since it was a double loop, I saw my dad and my brother many times. They were so excited for me. Tom ran alongside each time I passed, asking how I was, giving encouragement, and seeing if I needed anything. Second, the last time I saw Tom, he exclaimed that I was passing people. Funny, I don't remember that. During the last six miles, I felt very strong. I maintained a steady pace. Although I was frustrated at the beginning, I zoned out as the race progressed. Perfect—it was a nice boost to hear that I was passing others. Third, as I approached the finish line, one of the ladies I had eaten dinner with the night before was running alongside me, cheering. A near-total stranger was run-

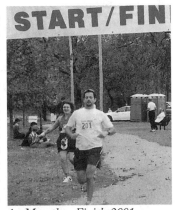

1st Marathon Finish; 2001

81

ning, with her arms raised, shouting encouragement to me. The exchange of encouragement between total strangers is beautiful to witness. The connection we feel to one another is one of those unique human qualities that helps me know I'm not alone.

It was amazing to me that my middle-of-the-pack finish could produce such a reaction. Later, I found a famous photo of marathon runner Jim Ryun finishing a race. I love this particular photo of Jim Ryun. The photo was taken at the very instant he finished a one-mile race; but this was no ordinary one mile. This was the first time in history that a high school athlete had finished one mile in less than 4 minutes. A world record had just been made, and the crowd was going *wild*. In the photo, you can see the last few feet of the race, and the onlookers are clapping, raising their arms, and cheering. The race official seems the most overtaken with joy, as he leapt into the air with his arms raised. What emotion!

When I put Jim Ryun's one-mile world record finish and my middle of the pack marathon completion together, I couldn't believe we could induce the same reaction. What I now know from comparing these pictures is that our joy is not confined to the elite few who will hold a record. It's overcoming odds that we delight in and share with one another, and you don't have to be a world champion to overcome odds.

My goal finish time was 4:21:00. The picture of me crossing the finish line is 4:21:00. In the 8 subsequent marathons and nearly 20 half marathons I have run, I have never hit my goal like that. My reaction in that moment was very matter-of-fact. My focus was on stopping my watch. My thoughts were these: I trained... I succeeded; this is what happens when you train properly and diligently. While that can be true, in endurance sports it's not always the case, as I would find out later.

Directly after the race, we took my brother to the airport, and Dad and I started the drive home. I didn't know how I would feel emotionally or physically after the race; I had never run 26.2 miles or trained for anything so hard and so carefully for so long. All I can say is that I'm incredibly thankful we took Dad's R.V. for the 8-hour drive home. If I could not have stretched out I think I would have died. I was in so much discomfort it was ridiculous; I literally couldn't move without something protesting. I swear one more step on the race, and my eyelids would've cramped after blinking. Pretty much that entire day after the race, I was sleeping, eating, drinking, or stretching. Emotionally, I felt relieved and excited. I was relieved that many months of hard work and achieving little goals along the way had paid off. I was relieved that my condition hadn't interfered with my preparation or race. I was excited to have finished at my time goal. I was excited because I had found a way to positively deal with a chronic illness.

My intention when starting this whole "running thing" was to improve myself. To become more constructive in my thoughts. Inspiring others was nowhere on my radar. Not that I was opposed to that happening—but it wasn't part of the plan. Sometimes you're in the right place at the right time doing the right thing, and unexpected good things happen on their own.

During the drive home, my father told me he had had a conversation with a spectator. No surprise there; Dad will strike up a chat with anyone. What was interesting is that he took a walk, a few miles into the course, and noticed a lone spectator. As he introduced himself, she asked who he was there with. When he told her, Dad asked her the same question and she answered that she was with her husband. She explained that her husband ran primarily to maintain his health. She returned the question, and Dad said something to the effect of "my son has a medical condition and this is what he does to stay healthy." Dad mentioned what my medical condition was, and the woman started crying. Her sister had three children with my disease and she had never heard of anything like this before. She was shocked and elated to know there were great possibilities for her nieces and nephews. She couldn't wait to call her sister and tell her about my father and me. I'm so glad my dad decided to stretch his legs, get a different view, and randomly stop and chat with a stranger.

Armed with a successful marathon, a new attitude, and the notion that there was some other purpose to this whole thing called life, I immediately started planning my next marathon! I could sum up my immersion in running as this: keep your focus on something positive, and the things you *have* to do... just may become the things you *want* to do.

Chapter 10

RUNNING FEVER

*"To give anything less than your best
is to sacrifice the gift."*

Steve Prefontaine, Olympic runner

I was officially hooked and wanted more. Some amazing physical effects happened to me as a result of my first year training for the marathon. First, I gained ten pounds. It is extremely difficult for someone to gain weight with my condition. The digestive enzymes secreted by the pancreas are blocked, so I must take over 10,000 pills per year simply to digest food. These are big, blocky pills, and they are loaded with synthetic digestive enzymes. The average person with my condition absorbs around 60% of the nutrients from the food they eat. You can quickly see why we are typically skinny. I choose the word *skinny* with purpose. Lean bodies are terrific, but skinny bodies indicate a problem. Gaining ten pounds while running 30 miles or so a week was truly unexpected.

My lungs were also clearer than they had been in years. While many people at my age are declining rapidly or outright dying, I was the healthiest patient at my clinic. The worst part of this condition, and the part that kills, is loss of lung function. People with my condition have unusually thick mucus in their lungs. Not to gross you out—but you know when you get sick and cough? You know how that stuff looks? (Green and yellow?) That's what my mucus *always* looks like. (That's right, super gross!) That thick mucus traps a whole host of nasty little organisms. Viruses and bacteria that don't stick around in normal lungs are trapped and grow in our lungs. This thick substance in my lungs is a breeding ground for some nasty and deadly bugs. The worst thing is that you can't avoid them; every time you turn on the shower, for example, you get a face full of these germs. To have lungs that don't sound like one has pneumonia is rare at my age, and to have clear lungs is unheard of.

Another aspect about me that changed during my marathon training was my attitude toward this disease and my life with it. I was no longer worried about dying young or suffering. I came to the realization that I really have no control over my body with this disease. The disease will do what it does, and while the medicine increases my chance of success significantly, there is no cure. I WILL get lung infections. Any one of those infections could be the infection that starts the process of multiple infections that leads to my death. I have heard stories of slow decline, of the disease taking years to overtake the body; I've also heard stories of my peers with this disease getting sick and dying within a matter of months. What I learned was that it didn't matter what *could* happen, but rather what I *made* happen. I could either spend my life worrying and trying to ignore my condition, or I could embrace the fight.

Embracing the fight or embracing the pain, as I call it, doesn't mean I go looking for trouble. Believe me, I have enough to be concerned about without making life harder. I'm only saying that if there *is* a challenge out there in front of me, I grab it and take a hold of it—or it will take a hold of me. By grabbing the challenge and getting my arms around it, I can work to get my *head* around it. Once I've got my head around the thing, I can find ways to overcome it. You know the old adage: keep your friends close, and your enemies closer. What this means is that by keeping your enemies close, you can easily watch them and be ready for what they do. I found this to be true when applied to my challenges. By being more in tune with how I felt physically and emotionally, I could act quicker to make changes. *Embracing* also means more than merely accepting. I accepted the fact that I had this disease through all those years before my 30th birthday. I had moved beyond denial, but I still didn't want to deal with the possible consequences, so I pushed it away as much as I could. Once I brought it closer and really started to embrace my life with this thing, I changed myself. By embracing the challenge and being comfortable with life, I was able to then reach out to others who needed encouragement. I also was able to truly be a spouse to somebody.

Upon completing that first race, I looked for the next one. This time, I wanted to have the "marathon experience." I wanted to travel to a "cool" city and run in a race with a good reputation. The best marathons are known for being organized, fun, and fast. I pretty well knew where my next race was going to be. Living in St. Louis, the obvious choice for me was the Chicago Marathon. A race with 50,000 other marathoners, a seriously cool town to visit, and a race course that attracted runners from around the world because it was flat and fast.

I discovered that I really wanted to beat my previous time. I was pretty sure this could be done, as I had energy to spare in Tulsa. I found a new training program and started up again. I ran a warm-up half marathon that spring and smoked it. Funny how quickly 13.1 miles had become a warm-up! Through early summer, I hit finish times that were all faster than the previous year's. This new training model was going to make this next race a piece of cake, I thought.

Then midsummer hit, and during the dog days I got slower. Still being relatively inexperienced, I was concerned about my lack of real progress between mid-June and mid-September.

Here in St. Louis, we get summer heat like the South. 90-plus degree days are quite normal. Like the South, we also get humidity. 90% humidity is very common. Heat and humidity make for miserable conditions to run in. Whether you get up at 4 AM or wait till 10 PM, it's still going to be over 80 degrees and 90% humidity. Welcome to Missouri!

I actually started to take pride in saying I got my training runs in during the heat, and it felt like a badge of honor. While I was immersed in a culture of "obsessed marathoners," secretly I was worried that my times were getting slower; by September 1st I only had a month and 2 weeks of training left. I was running more slowly and feeling worse at a slower pace, and my worry was growing. I asked other runners if my slowness was normal, and they affirmed that times get slower in the summer, and that it would be ok in the end. I sure wanted to believe them, but how do you just trust someone? I figured it was just another quirk of this ridiculous body of mine.

The summer temperature finally broke, and my speed jumped right back up. To my stubborn surprise, I was running faster than planned and not feeling fatigued doing it. It seems that in endurance training, there is always something you can count on to make the challenge harder. From bad weather to injuries to summer heat, some years it is simply a continual battle. Just as everything was seemingly going well, my hip started to hurt badly. Nothing helped except taking tons of ibuprofen. I learned later that this is one of those things that is really unwise, not to mention potentially dangerous to your health. We can get so focused on a goal that sometimes we forget what is good for us. Many runners, including myself, get so driven to run in a particular race that we throw all caution and common sense to the wind. Regardless of my hip pain, the race was coming up and I WAS going to Chicago. Besides, I was running so fast.

My hip did bother me during the race, and from Mile 13 on I fought the discomfort. Despite the pain in my hip it was quite fun to be looking at my watch knowing that each passing mile was faster than planned. My goal was to beat my first marathon, and I was well on track to do that. During this race I felt none of the fatigue a runner normally feels. Coming down that final stretch with thousands of spectators cheering me on, I was able to cruise to the finish with a bit of a kick.

I had returned to Chicago for *me*. I will never see the unbroken tape of a finish line. I won't even finish in the top ranks of my age group. Typically, in a large field of runners, I'm in the 40th percentile. But running the last several hundred meters in Chicago, with thousands of people yelling and screaming in the bleachers, made me feel like I was the first person to finish. When I looked at the finishing clock, I knew I had broken my personal record. I beat my first marathon by eleven minutes: I had crushed it! Once again, the many months of preparation and dedication to running every mile at every scheduled distance and speed had paid off. I was a year older with this disease, and I still ran faster and with less discomfort.

For Chicago, my father and my mother accompanied me. Dad even drove the R.V. again so I could shower and change before the trip home. Two other people were there as well: my two best friends. I had known Mike since the third grade, and I'd known his wife, Julie, since college. I was there when they first met and I was honored to be the best man at their wedding. Mike and I were the only guys left from our high school crowd that stayed in town for college, so we hung out quite a bit when everyone else was off at school. We hung out frequently after college until I moved to Colorado. During difficult times, they were quietly supportive of whatever I needed. After all my years away from St. Louis, and of all the places I could have bought a house upon my return to St. Louis, a house went up for sale right next door to them. Seems like an odd coincidence. Together, they have been a rock of friendship for twenty years. When I moved back to St. Louis and had to regain my health, it was Julie's self-appointed task to "fatten me up." (Perhaps that's where the 10 pounds during marathon training came from!) I can't tell you how many meals she fed me. To get me back in the swing of "home," they invited me to all their family functions. I felt as if I were an extension of their family. During that first unsettling year in St. Louis, I could always drop by and just hang out. That was very calming, and if Julie ever got tired of me hanging around, she never said so. I wish everyone could have at least one friend like Mike or Julie—and I've got them both.

Attacking my health head-on and training for running were changing my life significantly, and I could not get enough. Almost immediately upon finishing the event in Chicago, I had my next marathon in sight, and I continued training without pause.

More Fever Sets In

Feeling ever more confident as a result of the massive personal record set in Chicago, I got "marathon fever" in earnest. I became one of those nuts you so often see running in the snow and rain and in temperatures ranging from 10 degrees to 100 degrees. I went as far as buying "Yak Traks"™ which attach to your shoes and allow safe running in ice and snow. I had an outfit for every weather condition and took pride in using them on the worst weather days. Everything in my life was adjusted for running the next marathon.

This focus on running was also seemingly good for other

things in my life. The discipline was carrying through to my work and health. I had learned the optimum plan for my nutrition and a daily routine that would allow me to eat well, work hard, and get in plenty of exercise. With this running fever, I had found an excellent life balance. During this time, I started dating my future wife as well (more about her later in this book). Getting to know Rene was another good decision during this time of focusing on the right things.

The Chicago Marathon was in the autumn of 2002. Keeping in shape, I remained in training mode for Grandma's Marathon in Duluth, Minnesota. Grandma's would happen in June of 2003. You may be asking, why go to Duluth when you can go to so many beautiful cities in the U.S? Because the marathon was well organized and had the reputation of being a great race. I had total marathon fever and didn't care if San Diego was the same weekend, because Grandma's had one of the best race reputations in the country.

Grandma's was a fun race in a beautiful setting, running 20 miles along the Lake Superior coast on a cool, sunny day. Marathoners had taken over the little town of Duluth for the weekend. Everywhere we went, we could spot the runners. Before the race they were wearing their t-shirts from other races, and their cars were plastered with "26.2" stickers. They certainly looked the part. At dinner, you could easily spot the runners because we were all eating the same thing: pasta and bread. After the race you could spot them a mile away by their "marathon gimp" and the grin of pride one wears after finishing a hard-fought battle.

Progression

The Duluth race was a bit more difficult than the previous two. On race day I felt great and had a decent finish, although my finishing time was slower than those in Tulsa and Chicago. It was difficult because the course was very hilly, but it was also different because I was battling some kind of stomach issue. The entire winter and spring of 2002 and 2003, I was experiencing recurrent stomach pain. As the months went on, the pain grew in intensity. Much like the doctors did when I was an infant, Rene and I started experimenting with food. Take out spicy food. Take out fatty food. We tried different portion sizes, thinking perhaps that digestion was a problem. The doctor thought that

I was lactose-intolerant, so we cut out dairy. Nothing worked consistently. My pain was quite severe and sometimes lasted for days. The pain would sap my energy, and I did not want to eat or exercise. Finally, one day as I was making sales calls, I had to pull over in my car as I could not bear the pain any longer. Sitting in a parking lot, doubled over in extreme pain, I called a doctor to schedule tests right away. The doctor told me to cancel our upcoming trip to Colorado, because the altitude could "burst" my stomach. Immediately we started with an MRI, which showed nothing. The CAT scan showed nothing as well. When the pain still did not stop, the doctor took a peek at my intestines. The lower endoscopy showed eight ulcers. Ulcers? I wasn't particularly stressed at work. Rene was a great joy in my life and I was eating very healthy with the running training. What was causing this?

Because digestive enzymes are not secreted properly in my body, the acid levels in my intestines can get very high. Enzymes work in conjunction with acid to digest food, and without the proper level of enzymes, the acid just eats away at everything on its own. The fix was easy enough, and I immediately started on a twice-daily anti-acid medication. Two more pills per day. This wasn't the worst thing that could have happened, and we were relieved. We were quite ecstatic to know that my stomach was not going to burst, or something else equally horrific. What the experience did show us was that my body was still vulnerable to this disease's ravages. No matter what we did to take care of my body, the disease could progress—and it did.

Progression Bonus

My CAT scan showed an irregular look to my pancreas. At first the doctor thought it might be pancreatitis, but I wasn't showing all the symptoms, and we had found the ulcers, which explained the pain. My pancreas still looked odd, however, so the doctor prescribed some additional blood work. The medical staff also asked some questions about how my energy level was; did I feel any other pain or jitters at any time, etc.? In general I was feeling great, other than the gut-wrenching pain of ulcers. After a few days on the anti-acid, I was feeling no pain, so obviously their additional questioning piqued my curiosity. My blood work showed a higher than normal A1C. That's technical jargon for high blood sugar. They suggested I pay attention to how I felt in the morning and after meals. The next clinic visit showed higher blood sugar levels. *Diabetes!* Now that was a bunch of *#%@$*, if you ask me. I'd spent a lifetime worrying about my lungs getting infected and losing weight because I didn't digest food. Now, Doc, you're telling me I could die from some other life-threatening disease?

As incredulous as I was, the fact remained that I had diabetes. The onset of diabetes was caused by the disease I live with. The abnormal CAT scan of the pancreas actually indicated that I had a pancreas that no longer functioned. So... now I had to worry about going blind, having my feet amputated, my heart failing, or having a diabetic stroke. My whole life, the doctors had told me to eat whatever I wanted. Eat ice cream, it will fatten you up. Eat pasta, it will fatten you up. Eat and drink anything: it will fatten you up!

Fortunately, I had already started eating better as a result of marathon training, so that mental game was not too difficult. I was more concerned about the progression of this disease and what new challenges I was now facing. Running had become very important "mental therapy" if you will, and I didn't know if there were elite athletes who had to deal with diabetes and what adjustments they had to make. Was this going to end my ability to run marathons?

On the Jumbotron

Rene and I had our moments of frustration, anger, and anxiety because of what this new disease did to me, but it would not bring us down. We figured it was "just one more thing" and we moved on to take care of things the best we could. It did not affect my desire to continue running. Like turning thirty and seeing that I was already older than my life expectancy, this bump in the road called "diabetes" just made me more determined to do well.

I took a break from marathons in 2004 and just ran a couple half marathons. I was battling some recurring injuries and needed to reduce my mileage. The break from marathons turned out to be a good thing, as I was able to excel at the half marathon distance and gain some confidence. I was running half marathons very fast, and that showed diabetes was not getting me. By 2005 I wanted another marathon, and decided I would run in my hometown marathon here in St. Louis. Per usual, my summer was spent training; although during this training season, I wasn't obsessed about every mile. I relaxed a bit and allowed myself some easing on my diet. I even missed a few runs here and there. I was an old pro now, after two full marathons and a handful of half marathons. In addition, I wasn't going for a personal record—I just wanted to enjoy this one.

On a very warm day in September of 2005, the Lewis and Clark Marathon was held. I was familiar with the course, having run the half marathon previously, and was totally confident. I was so relaxed at Mile 4 that I started a conversation with another runner. We hit it off quite well for total strangers. We ran side by side past Mile 19. Somewhere between Miles 19 and 20, my body had other ideas about the day. In that short mile, I had to say goodbye to my new friend and slow down quite a bit. After climbing one bear of a hill at the 24-mile mark, I was spent. In the next two miles, I declined to the point that I was walking and cramping up. My hamstring would cramp, and when I pulled up to ease that cramp, my calf would spasm. When I tightened up from the calf muscle, my quad would seize up. Then my neck started up, and I was walking with my head tilted to one side trying to ease that cramp.

That year we finished inside an arena. That was especially exciting because the spectators would be right there, up close. It was really quite unique. As we ran around, or in my case, trudged around the parking lot of the arena near the finish, we were funneled into a large doorway. We could hear the crowd inside the building. We could also hear music pounding. For the past two miles, I had been battling cramps and was alternating between walking and running. With the arena entrance now in sight and the crowd in my ears, I felt that familiar jolt of energy all runners feel at the end. This is when you see runners "kick" their last effort and straighten up so they look good crossing the finish line.

I wanted to look good finishing too, so I took off my water belt and threw it to one of the volunteers. As I threw the belt, my torso seized up. My body was not ready for that motion and was already fragile from serious dehydration. When I reacted to the torso cramps, *everything* locked up. Neck, shoulders, quads, hamstrings. I went down in a heap just outside the arena. A volunteer came rushing over to see if I was ok; I was not. I told her to just help me stand up and that I could walk the 50 feet into the arena. So much for my grand entrance—but at least I collapsed outside the arena, where only a few people saw. As I walked into the arena the crowd was cheering, and I saw my mom, wife, mother, and sister-in-law. They all had tears in their eyes. I thought, *wow*, they really were inspired by my latest marathon effort. Little did I know that there was a camera outside the arena, capturing the final approach of the race. The crowd could see the very moment their runner was coming in. My collapse had been captured on the Jumbotron, and that is why they were crying. When I found out I was on the Jumbotron at my weakest moment, I started sweating all over again, this time from embarrassment!

Pursuing a difficult goal will provide triumph, and sometimes it will also humble you. It will also teach you to not take preparing for that goal lightly when it pummels you into the ground. This race wrapped up all those things in a nice, sweaty, cramped-up, and embarrassing package. When I think back on this "failure" of a race, I have pride. I take pride in the fact that Rene and I came together to overcome a new obstacle. At the same time, I felt humbled that I was able to move forward with my new way of thinking, even in the face of ulcers and diabetes, and participate in my hometown marathon. After that day, I never took my preparation for a race for granted again.

This race was the beginning of a trend. My times at the full and half marathon distances would be slower over the next two years. In late October of 2006, I ran the Chicago Marathon again, and in October of 2007, I completed the Marine Corp Marathon in Washington D.C. Even with proper focus and dedication throughout training, my times were slower with each race. In between these full marathons, I competed in several half marathons, again each time being slower than the last. Part of me chalked this up to simply getting older. By the 2009 season, I was 39 years old. A lot happens with the body between 31 and 39; perhaps I was just getting older, I reasoned. I wasn't totally convinced of that, though, because I had several running buddies who were 20 years my senior and running faster at their age. Either they were superhuman studs, or my own body wasn't doing so well.

Chapter 11

NOT GOING DOWN WITHOUT A FIGHT

"The bold will never look back on their lives and wonder what could have been."

Michael Patrick Burke

When we stand on the sidelines and cheer somebody on, our hope is that our words of encouragement will energize our audience. This cheering is certainly a good thing. Our intended audience does get a rush when hearing those encouraging words, especially if it comes from a friend or loved one. When times are tough, an encouraging word or knowing that someone is praying for you can make a tremendous difference in a person's attitude. We call that *fellowship*. Knowing you're not alone in this world makes a big difference. If we want to take fellowship to the next level, we actually get in the game with them. Our actions will most certainly affect our target audience a great deal more than our words will, and we get the added benefit of changing ourselves for the better.

As a pace coach for marathoners, I had the privilege of helping a few hundred runners achieve their goal. Training for months and months on end, there are many times when motivation gets low, or you're just plain old exhausted. In those times, it was awesome to be able to give new life to someone else's goal. When one of my runners would complain about a sore muscle, how hard it is to eat right, or some other general gripe, I would say: "Hey, when your lungs are at 80%, you can't digest food, and have to manage diabetes, *then* you can complain about this running thing being difficult!" Of course, I would say that in a joking manner so as to not make them feel bad, but there was truth in my statement. Most of the time, as they were expressing their sorrows, they would stop themselves and say something to the effect of, "Look who I'm complaining too; I've got nothing to complain about." It was always inspiring to me to help my runners, whether in big or small ways. There was one particular time that I helped another runner that stands out in my mind.

My wife had seen an old high school friend at many of the races in St. Louis and at track workouts. Whether it was a marathon or a 5K, Jason was always around. Jason is the kind of guy you just love to be around. He is one of those people that make you feel like you are the most important person in the world when he is talking to you. You know by his questions and enthusiasm that he is genuinely interested in what is happening in your life. He always has wonderful words of encouragement and you leave his company in a great mood.

He also happens to be a very driven runner. As we got to know him better, we found out he had run well over 20 marathons. Jason was really fast and dedicated to the local runners club. He was a true "elite" type runner, and as a "middle of the pack" guy, I was amazed by him. Knowing that he was so involved with the runners club, training teams, and racing, it was odd that all of a sudden we didn't see him around at races. He was not at the normal places we would expect him. He was not at the track for speed work. He was not at the St. Patrick's Day Run, and *everybody* goes to the St. Patrick's Day Run. Nobody knew where he was. He had inexplicably dropped off the radar screen altogether, and we were wondering where the heck he was. Finally, through the grapevine, we heard that he was very sick.

The next time I saw him, he was at the 2009 GO! St. Louis half-marathon. It was a rainy April morning, and I was leading a group of 20 or so runners in a pace group. I noticed Jason running just ahead of us. As we came up alongside of him, I tapped him on the shoulder; in typical Jason fashion, he was excited to see me. We quickly caught up on our lives and I learned why he had been missing. Just a few months previously, a tumor was found on his brain; doctors had rushed him into surgery and removed it. I also learned this was his first effort at racing after his surgery. Jason was not feeling confident that he could finish. He was still suffering from some motor skill setbacks that came with his brain surgery. He had spent the last couple of months rehabilitating and it was a bit premature for him to return to running. According to the doctors, it was certainly too early for him to be running a half marathon. When he asked if he could run with my pace group, I was honored because he was such a stellar runner. When he said he was worried and that he didn't think he could finish without my help, I told him to stay close and we'd keep an eye on him.

I was having a great run that day. We were keeping a faster-than-expected pace, and Jason was tucked right in with us. Somewhere around Mile 7 of the 13.1 miles, I started to struggle. My stomach was upset and my energy level was deteriorating fast. Over the next few miles I became slower and slower, and in my own physical struggle I lost track of Jason. Since I was having a bad day, I assumed that he was somewhere ahead of me, but I didn't really know. Around Mile 11, there was a good-sized hill. It wasn't really steep, but it was a long hill and strategically placed toward the end of the race so as to kick every runner's butt. I was struggling so much with my bellyache and fatigue that I began to walk. I had let down my pace team and felt very upset. Nobody likes having a bad race, but when you are leading others and don't succeed, it hurts ten times worse.

Physically and mentally beat, I decided to take a short walk break that turned into a long walk break. All of a sudden, I felt a tap on my shoulder. As Jason came alongside me, he gave me a simple "come on." The guy who I had helped for half the race was now returning the favor. Those simple words, his fellowship, and a little dose of competition got me going again. Now with just a mile to go, we really picked up the pace. We started passing all kinds of people. As we passed my parents with about a half-mile to go, I was looking terrible and Jason was all smiles.

We were side-by-side, pushing one another along. We finished very strong, passing dozens of runners and coming across the finish line together in a near sprint. What a great day! The day wasn't great because I had a great race; the day was awesome because I experienced camaraderie at its finest.

I'm Not Going Down Like That

Our experience together wasn't over, however. That summer, we both trained for a full marathon. The 2009 Lewis and Clark Marathon in St. Charles, MO was scheduled for September. Jason wanted to complete his return to running by finishing another full marathon. I was upset at such a poor showing at the half marathon that I wanted redemption! Per usual, I dedicated 18 or so weeks to training. I was confident with the times I was putting in, and on race day I was ready. It was a nice morning, albeit a bit warm. I was excited to be doing something only 1% of the population will do—successfully finish a marathon.

Throughout the first half of the race, I was on a record pace. Going through the time check at 13.1 miles, I was looking and feeling great. I was on target for another record day. It was getting hotter though, and the sun was beating down. At Mile 19, I was fatiguing fast. I was using up my hydration too quickly and had dropped my salt tablets somewhere along the way. I was hoping to just slow down a bit and cruise through the last few miles. I was anticipating the difficulty of this part of the race, but it was hotter than I had expected. The next two miles or so were in the sun with no shade. By Mile 22, I was walking—with no chance of picking up the pace. Every time I tried running, I would feel a cramp come on and revert back to walking. I'd been in this spot before and I wasn't looking forward to walking 4 miles, feeling sick to my stomach, suffering through a pounding "dehydration headache," and spending the next couple hours mulling over my mistakes.

As I continued to walk, I had an intense desire to simply quit. The combination of being passed by other runners who looked like beginners and ambulances rushing to pick up other runners was torture. It had turned out to be an unusually hot day, and runners were bailing out all over. At one point I saw the "SAG" (Support and Gear) vehicle picking up those who were dropping out. It is a runner's nightmare and a massive hit to your pride to be gathered up by the SAG vehicle, for that means you completely failed in your goal. While I took a bit of comfort from the fact that I wasn't the only one struggling, it was not an encouraging afternoon. It is so dejecting knowing that you failed at something you've worked very hard to do well. My worst thoughts during this 4-mile death march were the thoughts that my disease, coupled with diabetes, had taken too great a toll on my body. For three years my times had been slowing, so perhaps I simply wasn't able to do this kind of thing anymore. Those were sobering thoughts.

In middle of this "pity party" I came to the realization that today didn't matter. Sometime during the "Lewis and Clark Death March," I decided I would re-dedicate myself to running and finishing a strong marathon. I wasn't going to accept so easily that this disease had gotten the better of me. I was going to do another race, and do it as soon as was reasonable. In sheer defiance of my medical condition, I walked the final miles to the end in the worst time I'd ever finished.

The very next day after that sobering experience, I registered for the St. Jude Marathon in Memphis, TN. St. Jude was in early December, so I had a few months to gather myself and get strong. Little did I know that Jason had had an equally disappointing 2009 Lewis and Clark race. He finished behind me, which I would not have expected in a million years. He was worried that the brain surgery had affected him to the point that he could never again be a strong runner. In the end, neither of us accepted that kind of fatalistic thinking. We started running together in preparation for Memphis.

When possible we ran together, and when we couldn't run together we talked about our progression. Memphis had a reputation for being hilly, so on my 16-, 18- and 20-mile training runs, I hit the hills. This took every bit of enjoyment out of my running life. *I hate hills*. But if you're going to run a hilly marathon, you have to get strong by running hills. Our confidence was growing together. Each week, our times were right were they needed to be and our legs were strong. Our goals were getting loftier. I let myself think I could make a personal record, if the Memphis weather cooperated.

Redemption

Jason rode down to Memphis with my wife and I. There was a large group of runners heading down to Memphis from

St. Louis, and we were all anticipating a great time. The night before the race, we had dinner with nearly 30 fellow runners. My wife was competing in the half marathon with her sister and some close friends she had trained with over the past few years. Rene was also a pace coach for the training teams, so she got to know many wonderful people. When you spend hours running together, you quickly bond; her group was tight-knit.

Looking at the weather forecast, it was going to be a cold and sunny day. Perfect! Early on race morning, the temperature was in the low 30s. We bundled up and gathered at the start line. I kissed Rene for good luck and exchanged hugs and high fives with our friends. As the start drew near, we stripped off our extra clothes and Jason and I got toward the front after exchanging our own "manshakes." You know—macho handshakes. Bumping knuckles! Whatever you want to call it, we were pumped.

The first couple of miles were over in a blink of an eye. The worst of the hills were in the first 3 miles, and we blew up and down them like they were nothing. We were truly running fast, and each mile was well below our goal time. By Mile 8, I asked if we should slow down and be conservative, as we still had a long way to go. We agreed to keep pressing it until we felt some fatigue. I observed something funny about Jason during the race. At each mile mark he would surge ahead and be the first one to reach the milepost. (Sneaky son of a gun!) I found out later that he has a little competitive streak and that this behavior is common. I've got a bit of a competitive streak as well; so on this day I decided I surely wasn't going to let him take *all* the mile marks.

My strategy was to run without music until I needed a little pick-me-up and distraction. So at the 20-mile mark, I put on my headphones. Trying to run, turn on the player, and put in my earpieces was proving harder than I anticipated, so I told Jason I needed to walk for 30 seconds to get situated. I figured he would keep going, but no—he slowed down with me. We were in this together. The tough miles were clicking off and the feeling of fatigue at Mile 20 went away. Miles 21, 22, 23, and 24 were faster than Mile 20. Nearing Mile 25, I started feeling worn out. Jason beat me to the Mile 25 post and I had to walk through the water station. Jason once again slowed to walk with me. 1.2 miles to go, and we had run every step together. Somewhere between

Mile 25 and Mile 26, I couldn't keep up. He was looking strong, though, and I wasn't going to hold him back. Normally when your partner pulls away it feels devastating, but today I wanted him to make his comeback complete with a personal best. I told him it was ok and to crush it. I was so proud that he worked so hard and overcame his physical and mental challenges. Seeing him take off ahead didn't devastate me that day. It inspired me to keep pushing for my own personal best.

Coming into the last half-mile or so, there were a few twists and turns through downtown Memphis. In the midst of the tall buildings, I lost sight of Jason. As I came into the baseball stadium where the finish line was, I saw the time clock. *I would have a personal record.* I crushed my best time by 4 minutes. As I crossed the finish line, I saw Jason waiting to congratulate me. As we exchanged "bro hugs" of congratulations and confirmed our personal records, the realization of conquering our fears and achieving a goal was overwhelming. This was the fastest race I had ever run, and I had erased the last several years of declining times. Not only had this disease and diabetes NOT tackled me, but once again I had proven I was living well.

Perspective

Rene had finished the half marathon before I finished my race. Ever my biggest cheerleader, she had been waiting for me at the finish. Having had such a great day and seeing Jason have a record day, I was really looking forward to hear how Rene, Brigit, Jackie, Dorothy, Kevin, and the other 30-some people from St. Louis had performed. There would be no time for that, however; when Rene approached me, she had an urgent message and we had to get back to the hotel right away.

Immediately after gathering my medal, warming blanket, and some food to recover, Rene told me that our friend Molly had also finished, but that she had been rushed to the hospital. Rene had coached Molly for a number of races. Over a couple of years, these two had spent countless hours together on the running trails. As I mentioned before, when you spend this kind of time together, great friendships are formed. A particularly special bond occurs as you go through the various trials and tribulations of endurance running. Molly was such a genuine person who was full of kindness and spirit, which attracted many people to her. Hearing the news that she had been rushed to the hospital was very alarming, as Molly had been diagnosed earlier that year with a heart condition. The diagnosis was surprising, as "the girls" had successfully run a series of half marathons for several years. Under doctors' orders, Molly dropped out of the racing scene, but was allowed to begin walking. The half marathon in Memphis was her first event since being medically cleared, and she had finished. While she wasn't pursuing a personal record, she was doing what connected her to her friends: staying healthy and completing a major goal.

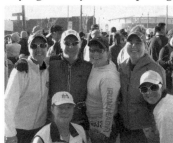

Memphis gang; Molly is on the far right, standing; Rene is the second in on the left

Not long after we were showered and changed, Rene's sister came to our room. The worst had happened; Molly had passed away. All the girls met at the hospital to support Molly's mother. (She was there to support her daughter and run in her first 5K. Molly had inspired her mom to run.) I could do nothing but stay in the hotel room and await further news on what was to happen. Instead of waiting helplessly, I took my Rosary to the nearest church and began praying for Molly, her family, and her friends. These prayers quickly led to a reminder of how precious life is; I was reminded that we should cherish those in our lives so much more and never take them for granted.

Molly's memory is an inspiration because she was fighting her fight with courage. She could have worried herself into doing nothing, but she wasn't like that. Molly was following doctor's orders and was taking charge of her health. She wanted to enjoy life, and that meant staying healthy and spending it with friends. We truly don't know when our time is up, and only the fearful will look back with regret. The memory of her embracing life keeps the St. Jude Memphis Marathon a positive page in my life's book.

Chapter 12

OPEN UP

"By not telling me you were in need, you denied me the opportunity to be your friend."

Art Snarzyk, St. Louis business coach

For a long time, I thought being a middle of the pack runner couldn't be interesting to anyone. I have to admit to myself that when I'm watching the Olympics, the Tour de France, or Ironman World Championships, I'm most interested in the front of the pack. Who's winning this thing and where is their competition? When I watch sports at all, I want to see what these men and women can do with God-given talents that I simply don't possess.

After completing a couple marathons, my mother said "let's get you on the news, because you're doing something special." I thought Mom was being Mom. (Of course she thinks I'm doing something special—I'm her baby and she is just proud of me!) My thoughts were along the lines of: *I'm just doing what I have to do to combat this disease.* Besides, I'm slow, I cough a lot, I pass gas much too often for cameras, and I don't even have the dubious distinction of being the last person to finish. I'm squarely in the middle.

Well, that kind of thinking apparently doesn't stop moms from telling the world about their baby boys (and girls). At least, it didn't stop *my* mom. She wrote off to every news station and newspaper in the St. Louis area, hoping to get some interest in my story. Mom is the best kind of person, not only because she was proud of me, but also because she wanted some greater good to come out of my efforts. Her idea was for me to get some "air time" to help raise some money for our cause. To my great surprise, I got a call from a local newspaper. A journalist came out to our home, and we had a wonderful time together. I liked him immediately, and what made it really awesome is that he was a runner as well. Steve knew exactly what it was like to try and eat right. It was not a stretch for him to imagine what it must be like to run while coughing hard enough to puke or running while your stomach is sore from severe cramping. What he did very well was understand and portray my fears, hopes, and attitude toward my disease. I was so excited when he asked if we could go running together. I was still confounded about why my story would be interesting to others, but if it could raise some money for a cause, I decided I certainly should open up.

The phone calls started coming in. Soon after Steve's story was published, writers from the *Post-Dispatch*, St. Louis's primary newspaper, called and we did yet another interview. Another well-told story was written. Basking in the glow of my newfound publicity, the biggest surprise came when one of the local television anchors called. Kay was impressed with my mom's short recounting of my life, and she wanted to learn more. You know—a "human interest story." By this time, I felt I was becoming an old pro! (Not.)

Kay brought her camera crew and some great questions. I felt comfortable working in front of cameras, but I was nervous because I wanted to do well for my cause and all the families who suffer from this disease. I really thought about my life and what running meant to me. I was ready to bare my soul for the first time. As it turns out, the story was aired, and once again the journalist portrayed my struggles and success very well. We were so happy to get some exposure for our fight against a terrible disease. I was feeling overjoyed that I could express my fears and hopes, and was hoping someone with my condition was watching. I never would have expected that in the following weeks, strangers would tell me that my approach to life made a difference in their own lives. Shortly after my TV story aired, I was running at my favorite park. Now, I run there 4 days a week, at the same time of day. I see the same people over and over, and usually we just nod a quick acknowledgment and continue on. The runner who passed me that day surprised the heck out of me.

I had admired Mike from afar. I knew a friend of his very well, and knew Mike was an accomplished marathoner and ultra-marathoner, and a good 10 or more years older than myself. Just so you know how impressive this guy is, an ultra-marathon means running for 30, 50, or 100 miles. Usually 50 to 100 miles is the norm. Can you imagine running 50 miles—and on top of that, on hiking trails? This guy was doing a couple of those a year *and* a couple marathons. And he wasn't just a middle of the pack guy like me; Mike was an animal. He was winning races constantly, and I thought it was fascinating that he was older than me and still showing us all how to do it. So when he blew by me at the park, it was no surprise—it was just another day of me eating his dust. It was a surprise, however, when he looked back. He looked back again, and then stopped running. He obviously thought he recognized me, but as I said, I admired him only from afar and we had not really been introduced. As I caught up to him, he started running next to me, and this was our conversation:

Him: "Are you Mike Burke?"

Me: "Uh, yes, you're Brian's friend, right?"

Him: "Yes. I saw your story on TV. You've inspired me, man."

Me: (Speechless)

Mike asked if he could run with me that night. My mind blown, again! I said sure—if he was willing to slow to my pace, otherwise we would have a very, very short run together. As we ran together, he began telling me how he was inspired by my story. He told me that he was an avid runner, but that this year had been really tough. He was struggling with soreness and injuries. He mentioned that he was considering stopping running, and then saw the news story. He explained that the story showed him that he could deal with his soreness and injuries if I could deal with dissipated lung capacity, inability to digest food, and living past my life expectancy. What could I say to that?

Having zero experience in that department, I just grinned and thanked him for sharing with me.

For years, I never wanted anyone to know about my struggles. I didn't want to show weakness. I didn't want to bring anyone down; I didn't want to be avoided or pitied. I didn't want to admit to myself that I thought a lot about dying at such a young age. Mike was asking a lot of questions, and for the first time I was telling someone about my life in a different way. In the past, if I would talk at all, I would keep things very light and try to paint a rosy picture. What I was finding out from a near-stranger is that I could express my fears and challenges and at the same time show him my hopes and dreams. Once people knew how difficult my journey was, and once they knew how hard I was fighting, the connection to hope was automatic.

We saw each other from time to time, but he is in another class of runners, so we lost contact for the most part. Through our mutual friends, I learned that Mike went on that year to finish a 50-mile race and a marathon. The marathon he finished qualified him for the Boston Marathon, which is very difficult to qualify for. He overcame his injuries and continued to run. Looking back, I am so amazed and humbled that I was a part of his journey. Our run together was a blip in our lives—40 minutes talking to a stranger and making a difference in each other's lives. Those 40 minutes changed how I thought about my life. I can only hope that 40 minutes meant half as much to Mike. That year, I heard from a number of people who saw my story and were inspired to continue their running despite their unique challenges.

I had viewed my life as a curse for so long. A life filled with tough decisions, limited options, and much suffering to come. This short run with Mike opened my eyes to a greater purpose to my life with this disease. For the first time, I could not only see why a slow, coughing, spitting, flatulent runner could be meaningful to others, but I could also see where my life fit into a larger puzzle of fellowship; and more importantly, how the telling of my life's story could contribute to something greater than myself.

I would not be bashful ever again about sharing my life with others.

Chapter 13

WIDE OPEN

*"If all you share is misery...
then all you'll get is misery."*

Michael Patrick Burke

I was beginning to understand why people were interested in a slow, "mediocre" runner. I looked at the athletes I admired. Some of them were tremendously gifted athletes, but others were not. What my most admired athletes had in common was that they maximized what they had and fought very hard to be in their profession. I think of Rocky Blier, a football running back with the Pittsburgh Steelers, who was severely injured in Vietnam. He returned to the States with excruciating pain, eventually regained his position, and was part of one of the greatest NFL teams of the 1970's. The other athlete I admire is a little guy. (No surprise there, right?) Along with the disadvantage of a small physical build, the "experts" said this guy was not gifted with great baseball talents. He did, however, work hard to overcome his lack of physical gifts. David Eckstein was part of two World Series Championship teams, as well as earning a

World Series MVP honor. Not bad for a guy who isn't "gifted!"

These two guys are great and give me great perspective when competing, but there is a certain group of athletes that make me cry every time I see them. These athletes are the hundreds of competitors in the Kona Ironman Triathlon that have overcome serious challenges in life. Many of them don't even finish the race, and that draws me ever more close to them. Every time I watch the televised Kona Ironman, I can't turn off the tears. It's a bit embarrassing, because my wife is usually watching with me. I'd feel bad, but I catch her wiping away her own tears *every time*. I'm so impressed with these individuals. I don't cry because they did or didn't make it; I get emotional because they had the guts to attempt such a daunting feat. That's what reaches to the deepest part of me.

We "get" struggle! We like to see our fellow humans take suffering and pummel it into ashes. Those that run away don't inspire us. Even more to the point, we are inspired by those that face adversity and conquer it. I began to realize that *that* is why anyone would care about an average runner who will never win a race. I'd be lucky to get into the top 30%. Realizing that my story resonated with others gave me courage to continue sharing my story with those who need a little encouragement.

Life is full of surprises, and in middle of all this marathon running and new publicity, a wonderful opportunity came up. My local running store started a training program. They wanted to help runners achieve their goals of completing a half or full marathon. The owners of Fleet Feet Sports in St. Louis wanted people of all ability groups to have the joy of finishing an endurance event. Now I stress *all* abilities, because guess who they asked to be a coach? (Yes that's right.) They needed a middle of the pack runner to coach other middle of the pack runners. I really couldn't believe I was being asked to take part in this. The first question I asked was "Why me? You know I'm pretty slow." I was hoping that they might say something to the effect that I was, in fact, an excellent runner, but that wasn't to be. Their response struck a chord with me that I hadn't really thought about. The point they made was that I had a great attitude and love for running. Most importantly, I knew what it was like to dedicate myself to a goal like a marathon or half marathon. In addition, the very thing that made me slow (this disease) was the one thing that made me understand the struggles these people would go through over a 12- or 18-week training cycle.

Little did I know that the people I would coach over the next 5 years would give me more encouragement and support than I could imagine giving to them. When you run together every week for 18 weeks, you get to talking. We were running every Saturday for anywhere from 1 to 4 hours together. That's a lot of time to get to know your running group. As we learned about one another, they would hear my own story of living with a deadly disease, and they soon became my biggest cheerleaders.

When I apologized for coughing, they would tell me they didn't notice. When I was having a rough day of running, they were worse than my mother with their questions: "What did you eat?" "Did you take your medicine?" "How's your blood sugar?" "Have you been to the doctor lately?" They were constantly asking how I was doing and took a genuine interest in my progress as an athlete. What was further amazing to me is that they found my running resume impressive. I was learning more about why they admired an average running resume, and I began to realize I wasn't living with a curse at all.

The greatest thing we learned together is that *struggle is good*. The aches, the pains, and the days you didn't feel like running. The days you could barely finish. The days you didn't finish. The 4 AM Saturday and Sunday mornings. The 100-degree heat. The awful-tasting sports supplements. It was all difficult, and yet we did it with joy. We complained to one another until it started to sound like real complaining. Then we would stop and remind each other how great the struggle was and to keep the goal in mind. Then the complaining would turn to bragging: "I can't believe we ran in that hurricane." We would reminisce about that day in January when we ran 10 miles in 10-degree temperatures, and how our beards and eyelashes froze with icicles. How we couldn't drink from our water bottles because they had frozen. Our entire struggle was awesome, and it was building something in us that nobody could take away. We were the "One Percenters!"

With each new training session, there was a new "batch" of runners that heard my story. I was no longer hesitant to share my challenges in life, mostly because my fellow runners taught me that it wasn't about struggle as much as it was about accomplishment. I loved hearing everyone's stories of why they had started running. Sometimes it was a simple goal, such as running a half marathon before turning 40. Others ran because they wanted to get in shape for their daughter's wedding and had become hooked; they'd been bitten by the "running bug."

An Every-Day Decision

Of all the stories, Mike's caught my attention the most. A few weeks into a new training session, Mike was running alongside me. Coach Leslie was leading the group, so Mike and I were just hanging out in the back. Very quietly, Mike told me he had something to share. It seemed a bit strange, the way he was being so secretive. (I thought he was going to say he was an ax-murderer and to watch out when we got to the woods!)

Instead, he told me he used to weigh 400 pounds! I didn't put him near 200, so I was blown away by his news. He shared how he had gained and lost weight over the years, but nothing kept him motivated. Finally, he realized that if he didn't keep the weight off, he would most likely not see his kids grow up. I asked how he had done it. Surely he had had one of those surgeries to reduce his stomach or he had loaded up on weight-loss pills. Nope. Mike began by simply walking around his neighborhood and completely changing his diet. Was it easy? Heck no! It is not one bit easy to make a life-changing decision and stick with it.

After some time and much determination, he had lost over 200 pounds. As would be expected, his confidence had grown, but his dedication was wavering. In order to keep focused on maintaining weight loss, he signed up to run a half marathon. There we were, two guys battling for very different reasons, but finding something inside us that we had in common. I liked him very much and respected his efforts. He had to *choose* to want something different. There was nothing like pain or something acute, like a heart attack, driving him. Mike just wanted something better and made the decision to do it. He has now completed many half marathons and at least one full marathon, and is one of the strongest and most lean runners I know.

Mike continues to encourage me, touching base often and asking how my running is going. If I'm slacking, after we talk I feel like a slug and get motivated again. Thanks, Mike.

Hurricane

Mike would not have it so easy for his first attempt at a half marathon. He dedicated himself to the many months of training, like everyone else. He suffered through the hot summer days and humidity. He ate well and learned all he could in order to have an excellent race. What he could not prepare for was Hurricane Ike. While you live in the Midwest, you get quite a bit of weather coming from the Gulf of Mexico. The Gulf weather comes right up the Mississippi River valley and usually socks us with heat and humidity. In September of 2008, Hurricane Ike was raging in the Gulf of Mexico and started tracking our way. For days, emails and calls were flying about what would happen if that hurricane came through St. Louis. Marathons *don't* get canceled; maybe delayed a bit, but NEVER canceled. During our training, we ran when it was raining. That might happen on race day, so it was good preparation.

Each day closer to the race, it was clear that we were going to get nailed by Hurricane Ike. Of course, it would be a tropical depression by the time it hit St. Louis, but they were forecasting up to 8" of rain in a half-day's time. In St. Louis, we do get downpours from thunderstorms, but not hours and hours of driving rain. I was hoping by some miracle that the training team would not have to show for the race. I'd already competed in enough races that I didn't need this extra "badge of courage."

As the morning of the race rolled around, the weather alarms went off. At 4:30 AM it was raining like crazy. We turned on the weather report and there was no hope of a break. It *was* going to be raining hard, but the race must go on. We called the training team director and were assured that the race was starting and that we were to be there. As we pulled into the parking lot near the starting line, the rain had already flooded the area. We had a Jeep and were not worried about the car. Our shoes and socks, however, were going to be soaked. Have you ever walked around in a wet pair of shoes and socks? Disgusting, right? Your feet get soaked and turn white and wrinkly. That day, our feet got soaked with our first step out of the car.

I was still hoping that the runners in my group would not show. After all, who would dare to run in that weather? Apparently, everyone! Every last runner from my pace group was there and chomping at their bits to get going. After a long delay, every part of us was soaked to the core. The veterans brought trash bags to wear and stay dry while the rookies got soaked to the skin before starting. It didn't matter though. Eventually, I had to shed my trash bag; I was instantly drowned. We might as well have been in a swimming pool. The rain was as thick as smoke. You couldn't see very far in front of you because the downpour was so heavy. Fortunately it was a warm rain, and once wet and concentrating on running, I forgot about it. Mike was totally excited to be doing this race. Nothing short of a tornado would have stopped him from running.

As we clicked off the miles, we were running fairly fast. The rain was keeping us cool and there were no heavy winds to fight. Mike and a couple other runners in my group picked up the pace, so he was having a good race despite the weather setback. After crossing the Missouri River, we were close to the halfway point. Coming down the exit ramp off the highway, I noticed that the volunteers were redirecting runners to the opposite direction of the expected route. My guess was that the roads along the river that we were scheduled to take were flooded. I quickly calculated: 3 miles or so would have to be made up from our diversion, depending on the total closures ahead. Someone heard a volunteer say we were only going to run 10 miles because trees had fallen over our path and the streets were flooded.

This started to sink in with the newbies, and in particular with Mike. He had dedicated well over a year to losing weight, changing his lifestyle, and training like a madman for this race. When we caught up with each other at the end I was trying to make him feel better, but there was no consolation. He knew it was nobody's fault, and that realization probably made it worse in the short run. Sometimes stuff just happens that we can't control, and knowing that you have no control over the situation can make it feel worse. Mike learned that sometimes you just take what is given and make the best of it. Still, not completing 13.1 miles that day did not discourage him. By November he completed his first half marathon with flying colors.

We didn't just make the best of running in a hurricane—we *reveled* in it. We made t-shirts that said "I Ran With Ike." I wear that shirt with pride and often think that if I had not been coaching during that time, I would not have had such a unique and memorable experience. I'm so happy that I opened up and shared my story to these runners. I'm so grateful they let me in on their own secrets as well, because they continually inspire me. I never once felt like my runners were complaining about the challenges they faced. I really liked the attitude of "the conqueror" that they were developing or had already developed.

I never sensed that these people were running away from their problems or challenges. They had picked a very constructive and healthy tool to conquer and destroy whatever personal obstacle was holding them back.

Being totally immersed in the culture of these runners helped me to gain a constant source of support. They also pushed me to go further and faster. You couldn't be negative for too long with these people. It just wasn't in their DNA to be a bummer. I could be real with them, and they in turn could be real with me about their challenges—it was a wonderful reversal of the old adage "Misery loves company." For us, *victory* loved company!

Chapter 14

IN THE FIGHT

*"Learn from the mistakes of others.
You can never live long enough
to make them all yourself."*

Groucho Marx, American comedian and actor

Of Hollywood Stars...

I wish I were half as good-looking as George Clooney is. It just so happened that the famous actor was in St. Louis shooting a movie at the same time our training team was part of a documentary also being filmed in St. Louis. So I'm sure the mistaken identity was a combination of cold weather, clothing, a beard, cameras following our running group, and plenty of distance between myself and the person asking the question.

What started the confusion that day was a van pulling alongside my little group of runners. The van doors flew open and from within the van a camera zoomed in on us. For a brief second, I was expecting a bunch of clowns to come tumbling out of the van—but it was just a film crew. The crew was getting footage during a cold day of running for the PBS documentary *Start to Finish: Running the Go! St. Louis Marathon*. It was one of those cool moments in life when you ask, "How did I get here?"

Well, I got to that moment mostly because I have a life-threatening disease. If I didn't have this disease, I probably would never have appeared in a documentary, much less been one of its featured stories. Without this condition, I sometimes question if I would have any drive to run marathons at all. And if I did run marathons, there would be nothing to separate me from the millions of other runners completing the 26.2-mile haul. Apparently, I was "a good story."

The documentary was really about the preparation needed for a major endurance race. The documentary took a look at race directors and athletes during the many months of training and planning. When the film crew asked the organizer of the training team if there were any good stories inside the "main" story, my name came up. As I've already mentioned in previous chapters, there are three major obsessions with endurance athletes: lung capacity, nutrition, and hydration. With my body acting in ways counterproductive to all three of those factors, plus the "bonus" of diabetes, I was one heck of a running story.

For most normal bodies, 26.2 miles is a challenge. With my body not digesting food, processing oxygen poorly, and losing electrolytes at alarming rates, the crew knew they had a unique story. By now, I was more than OK with sharing my once-private thoughts, fears, and hopes. When the filmmaker asked if I was willing to be interviewed and followed for 12 weeks, I jumped at the prospect. I really wanted people to see how difficult it was to manage life with this disease—I wanted to share how hard it was, yes, but at the same time to let the film's viewers see that there is a better way to live than to merely stand on the sidelines of one's life.

The filmmaker and crew interviewed me before training started. They followed my group with cameras every Saturday. They came out to my house to interview my wife and myself. They visited my parents to interview them. (On a side note, my dad talked so much they actually ran out of film.) Finally, they filmed us on race day. After many hours of footage had been captured, they went to work editing. Many months later the film was ready; the big release day was announced and our training group leaders put together a "viewing party." There were a ton of us crowding in to watch the premiere.

It was weird seeing my face and hearing my voice on a television. Not because I thought I looked bad or sounded odd—I just couldn't get my mind around how this had all come about. How did I get put in the same documentary with a cancer survivor and a runner who suffers with the excruciating pain of arthritis? How am I worthy of being in their company, and what about the scores of runners who have it worse than me? I was truly honored and proud to be a part of the film. The filmmaker, Anne Marie, did an incredible job telling our story. What I was most hoping for, deep down, was that somebody with my condition would see the film, be encouraged, and at least see through the blinding limitations of their condition.

A Connection

A few months after the documentary was released, a woman visited the directors of the training team. She knew from the film that I was somehow involved with them, and she asked if I worked in their stores. The staff at Fleet Feet told her I didn't work there, but could probably get us in contact. Trying to be safe, the staff asked who she was and why she wanted to talk to me. As they learned, this woman had a daughter who was recently diagnosed with my disease. She had seen the documentary and wanted me to speak with her daughter. That fact alone would have given her enough urgency for us to touch base, but the shocker was still to come.

This daughter (who had recently found out she had this condition) was diagnosed at 40 years old! Remember, this is a genetic disease and the overwhelming majority of those living with it are diagnosed as children. The average life expectancy was barely over 30. To find this out at 40 is rare indeed. Can you imagine what it is like to be told at 40 that you have a killer disease? To make it more devastating, at 40 you are already beyond the life expectancy. The shock of the diagnosis was taking a huge physical and mental toll on her family. The woman with the condition had daughters of her own, and that caused additional stress.

Well, Grandma wanted me to talk to her newly diagnosed daughter. This was not going to be fun. Nobody likes Mom meddling in his or her life, and Mom had just meddled big time. I could hear her: "A stranger is going to call me?" "What, and give me some advice?" I was nervous, but yet not scared to make that phone call. I wanted to be helpful, but really had no experience in such matters. I boiled it down to hoping to say the right words, *not* say the wrong words, and listen. (Not easy for this talker.) When she answered the phone, I introduced myself as the man with her disease who had been featured in the documentary. I reminded her that her mom had asked me to call. She responded in an annoyed tone: "I know who you are." I let her know I understood that she really might not want to speak to me. I told her it would be hard for me, diagnosed as a young child, to totally understand how it must feel to be her. I simply told her: if you have ever had thoughts of feeling alone, sad, frustrated, or desperate, we've experienced the same things. I also mentioned that if she'd ever had thoughts of not wanting to be a burden, or didn't want to think about "it" or take all the prescribed medicine, we'd also been in the same place. I gave her my phone number and said: if you feel or think those things, give me a call. Do you have any questions?

Apparently, I'd hit the mark. We ended up speaking for quite a long time. She was downright terrified of dying and leaving her daughters alone. She was paralyzed by fear and her health was getting worse rapidly. Untrained and inexperienced doctors were giving her the wrong medical treatments and telling her the worst things about her life expectancy. I desperately wanted to do something, but I was now really nervous and afraid of a blunder. I figured something about "being in the trenches together" would help out. I began by sharing my own life, living with this chronic illness. I started with my struggle of doubt and fear as a young adult. Then we talked about the avoidance and bad decisions that affected my health as a twenty-something. We talked about the first time I lost significant lung capacity. She seemed to understand and empathize with my life-long journey. The big difference between us was that the journey that took me a lifetime was taking place in her life at a rapid-fire pace. I had years to come to terms with my body; she did not have that kind of grace period.

I didn't want it to turn into a mutual pity party, so we started talking about some positives. I pointed out that she was so healthy all those years that she didn't even know she had this disease. Maybe her genetic mutation wouldn't cause as much trouble as it does for those who are affected much younger. We discussed how visiting a specialist could possibly make all the difference in the world. Not only was she not taking all the medicine she should—she was actually being prescribed counterproductive medicine. We talked about how much her mom loved her, and how special it was for her to have two daughters of her own. I assured her that life was beautiful and that although this disease could be a real son of a gun, she didn't have to let it rule her thoughts in a destructive way.

After a long time on the phone, I emphasized what her mother had done. While her mother had overstepped some boundaries, she was desperately trying to help, and all that meant is that she loved her daughter greatly. I reminded her that her daughters were watching her struggle. They were learning lessons about how to fight in life. I let her know how difficult it was to be forced to sit on the sidelines and watch a loved one fall into despair. We talked about how unfair that pressure can seem, but also about how uplifting it can be to inspire the ones so near and dear to you.

That was the moment I truly appreciated what my parents must have gone through those many years; the years I was away from home and their knowing I wasn't going to the doctor regularly and that I was losing weight and getting sick. As we continued to talk, I felt she was coming around to a better place. She wanted to hear some good news, and I was able to give her a bit. I really wanted her to contact my own specialist, because she could make some simple changes under his guidance and feel much better. We agreed that if I made an appointment with him she would consider going.

When I next spoke to my doctor, I gave him the summary of her entire situation as I knew it. Her current doctor knew very little about her condition and was not only missing treatments, but was recommending treatments that were counterproductive. I requested that my doctor didn't grill her about her current state of medications and therapies. I reminded my doctor how difficult this must be for her and that we should move forward in giving her true hope and guidance for her future health. Upon calling my new acquaintance back and giving her the appointment details, she was not enthusiastic. I honestly didn't know if she would go to the doctor at all. I asked her to call me back after her visit. With HIPPA rules prohibiting my doctor from telling me if he'd seen her, I would never know what happened unless she called me. A couple weeks went by after her scheduled visit and I heard nothing. My hopes of being a good listener and sharer of a hopeful message were waning.

I can recall just what I was doing that day when my phone rang. I was distributing some fliers for my business; it was a gorgeous day with the sun shining. I was on the front porch of a house and when my phone rang. I walked to the street to answer. Her voice sounded excited and confident. She had gone to the doctor's appointment, and oh my gosh, did they have a different story to tell her. In addition to prescribing new medicines and therapies, they told her she was not, in fact, going to die tomorrow. She was not doomed to die this year or the next. If she would take the medicine, do the therapies, and watch her health, she could likely live quite well for a very long time. The joy in her voice was a real gift. I had made a difference.

That kind of intimate experience with a fellow sufferer had never happened to me before. Yes, I had given speeches and been on the news, and people had expressed how my story inspired them in some way. While that still astounds me, this woman was something altogether different. I, first hand, had made a difference in somebody's life. The unique experience of living with a deadly disease had allowed me to reach out to someone. For the first time in my life, I could say I understood that suffering could produce good things.

I wish I could say she has overcome her fears and struggles. I've checked in with her a time or two, and she has since been forced to quit her job because her condition is getting worse. Taking medicine and doing therapy seems futile to her at times. I may have run the course of what I can do for her. I hope she continues to open her mind to the great gift she has in life and in the lives of her daughters. My hope is that she will let go of sadness and appreciate what she has right now.

Every time I tell this story, I realize that her life has great purpose beyond our understanding. I tell this story to remind others that they need to extend help and understanding to others. We need to extend ourselves, even when it is difficult to do so. *Especially* when it is difficult. We never know who will hear us, see us, or hear about us. When we fight our personal battles well, we inspire others. That is a very great privilege.

Chapter 15

THE GIFT OF WOMEN

*"Gentleness can only be expected
from the strong."*

Leo Buscaglia, author and motivational speaker

I am now going to digress a bit from my marathon stories, because I feel it is very important to tell my readers about the most important influences and supports in my life: the women I have known. I have to give special recognition to the great women that have shown me the way and shaped me into the person I am today. In my youth, I underestimated the capacity for love and strength that was shown to me by a wide range of women, and I hope in my more-mature years that I am able to "make it up to them." If I had been more in tune with my mom, her friends, my girlfriends, and simply "girl friends," I think I could have eased my fear of being alone much earlier than I did.

My Greatest Fear

Remember that my greatest fear as a youth was that no woman in her right mind would want to be involved with me, or would be strong enough to handle life with a chronic illness. Interestingly enough, as a teenager, this fear was far greater than the fear of dying. Looking back with the clarity that hindsight brings, I guess that makes sense, as kids primarily want to fit in and be accepted. I had convinced myself that no woman would ever invite me into her life.

The life expectancy number wasn't the only scary aspect of my condition. There literally were no adults with my condition that I could look up to, see that they were doing well, and reassure me that everything could be okay. Searching for advanced-age survivors was just too much to hope for. Adults with my condition were so rare that the medical community had no adult-care programs. I received care at a pediatric hospital until I graduated college. Adult care programs were founded when there were enough adult survivors alive to justify it. I had the unique distinction of being a part of the first generation to survive into adulthood with any significant numbers. These circumstances would surely create hesitation in a future spouse's mind. Adding insult to injury, one of the side effects of my condition is the inability (except in rare cases) to have children. I would be denied one of God's most precious blessings. I wasn't the most sensitive or child-oriented guy, but I came from a family of four brothers and it was natural for me to want children in the future. On top of all the other issues, I saw the inability to father children as the final obstacle that would chase ladies away.

Earlier in this book, I alluded to my missing clues about women... particularly during my interactions with my friend Katrina. What I should have recognized was that women were not only capable of handling this disease in their lives—they also wouldn't be repulsed by it. What I should have seen is that women are loving, caring, compassionate, and a lot stronger than I could comprehend as a teenager. If only I had seen the signs earlier...

Melissa

In 1990, I was a junior at the University of Missouri - Columbia. Upon entering my first college German class, I sat next to a beautiful girl. We got to know each other a little bit, but like all funny, smart, and beautiful girls, she, of course, had a boyfriend. The following semester we would see each other nearly every day, as our German II classes were back-to-back and in the same classroom. It became customary for us to greet each other in German. I spoke only four words to her every day for the next several months: *guten morgan*, Frau Meyer. That was it; four words. As we entered final exams, we found ourselves studying together and getting to know each other. We began dating shortly thereafter.

I talked to Melissa about my condition. She did her own research and was seemingly unfazed by it all. That summer I would go into the hospital for another "tune up." It should not have shocked me that she would want to visit me in the hospital, but it did. I was amazed that she would drive four hours from her home in Kansas City to where I was hospitalized. Seeing me in the hospital, in that state, with IVs hooked up and all, I knew would be a real test for her. She knew the symptoms, required medicine, and general outlook of my condition. She had spoken to her family about the condition and what it meant. While her sister was cautious and challenged her to think about what life would be like if she were to choose long-term plans with me, she and her family were more than willing to embrace me. I fell in love like an anvil falls from a window. We dated during our last two years in college and were married one month after she graduated.

Unfortunately, our marriage would not last. I can't speak for Melissa, but I know that I hadn't truly considered what it would mean to live with another person, especially with this medical condition hanging over our heads. We lived far from our families and I had a demanding job. While working long hours, my health started to decline. With so many unanswered questions, and, at least on my part, an unwillingness to communicate meaningfully, we had our handicaps from the very beginning. Staying together because we had feelings of love was not enough. We were not living with the other as our priority.

Getting married to your best friend is a great start, but staying together through the everyday grind of marriage, and then getting through major challenges, requires a best friend plus a whole lot more. Something stronger than friendship was needed, something that has at its core a constant reminder to help us communicate, forgive, move on from hurts, and always keep the other half as a priority. We didn't understand what being a best friend PLUS meant. By the time I was willing to talk openly about my medical condition and how it affected us, it was too late. She had willingly come into the fight with me, but watched for too long my not taking medicines and not doing the necessary therapies. Along with the stresses of job changes, moves away from family, and the challenges of my disease, we were selfish. We were simply not ready to be a team and sacrifice for one another to accomplish great things together.

From the experience, however, I learned that I *could* have a great woman in my life. I also learned that a great woman would jump in with me with both feet. Ultimately, I came to understand that I had a huge responsibility to do everything possible to ensure my good health. I needed to fight hard for my health, because it's just too difficult for a partner to sit on the sidelines and watch the person they love most losing interest in taking care of himself or herself. Attending to my health would be the very least thing I could do for anybody who would willingly accept a life that was all but guaranteed to have great challenges.

The Many Mothers I've Known

Growing up, I was blessed with many friends, and like most kids, we spent many nights at each other's homes. Each Friday our fathers would play softball, and during many of those games, we strategized about where we should spend the night... often based on who had the best food or the best toys. We would then beg and plead with our parents to ensure our overnight adventure would happen.

Imagine being a young mother and inviting a child into your home. Imagine that that child must take lots of medicine or suffer serious consequences. Consider this mother taking on the responsibility for the health of someone else's child. I dare say it would make most moms quite nervous. The easy road would have been to be overly cautious and, with all the grace one could muster, not invite that child to stay overnight. My parents were incredibly fortunate to have known several very special couples.

As my parents tell it, nobody cared. Yes, each mother wanted to know what the regimen was. Some needed more details than others, but all these women were comfortable in the fact that I was self-sustaining and I knew what I needed to do. None of them, however, let me slide on taking my medicine. Just like my mom, these great women didn't single me out or make me feel different. If they were nervous, they never showed it.

When I see these women today, my heart warms and I still

feel like a kid in their presence. When I get a hug from the Judys, Barbs, Nancys, or any of the other moms I grew up with, I feel their genuine care for me. Their first question is always "How are you doing?" This is no ordinary greeting born out of obligation, but rather their genuinely caring nature wanting to know if I'm doing well (like I'm one of their own). This is just how those families are, and I hope everyone has the privilege of "alternate moms" like these.

"Moms Away from Mom"

I moved away from home to see the world before my time was up. At times, I lived nearly 1,000 miles away. Though really not that far, it seemed like a huge leap back then. I loved being on my own, and my career progressed quickly. I began working a ton of hours but loved every minute of it. Finding time to visit home was not easy, since I worked most weekends and holidays. I was thrilled if I managed to get back once a year at Christmas. My mom naturally worried about me during that time. I did, however, have some other motherly souls looking out for me when I was away from my own mom.

Moose: Yes, I befriended a woman nicknamed "Moose." We worked together and she witnessed firsthand the aftermath of my divorce. She was quite a bit older than I was, and during that turbulent time, she was a calming presence. As she was no more than 100 pounds soaking wet, I don't know how she got that nickname. Perhaps it reflected her zest for life. She had run marathons and climbed "fourteeners." (Mountain peaks that are 14,000 ft. high or more.) She told me all about her adventures with the marathons in Anchorage and Pikes Peak. She was the first marathoner I ever knew, and she really piqued my interest in running and hiking. Moose and her husband, Rick, took me in as if one of their own. The first Thanksgiving I couldn't make it home, I spent with these two special people.

Linda: A genuine Southern woman; gentle, soft-spoken, smart, and full of fire... not someone to mess with. I met her when I moved to Virginia. Linda was my boss's assistant, and yet so much more. The company couldn't pay her what she did for our team in Richmond. Everyone leaned on her for support to get things done during our workday, and I leaned on her for moral support. Our hotel in Richmond was struggling when I arrived. It was a stressful environment, and as the assistant to the

Director Of Sales, Linda got the pleasure of hearing everyone's complaints. She wasn't in a position to make changes, but she genuinely listened to each of us. One day, a VIP guest of mine had a terrible experience. This guest, who had major influence on our revenue, was responsible for a big chunk of my bonus; so I was stressed, to say the least. I marched into Linda's office and told her (in a rather worked-up manner) about the issues that had cropped up. For some reason I was making it "personal" with her. During my diatribe, she put up her hand; I stopped immediately. Before kicking me out of her office, she gave me some "friendly" advice: she had a few choice things to say to me about respect and teamwork (and finding a girlfriend), because I was way too crabby to work with. With her Southern drawl, motherly qualities, and "I don't take any bull from anybody" attitude, I was enamored with her immediately. I laughed, apologized, and got the heck out of her office. For the next year and a half, she was my "mom away from mom." Linda sensed when I was stressed out and would insist we do the proper Southern thing—go have a cocktail at the swanky restaurant across the street to blow off steam. If she heard me coughing, she demanded I go to my doctor. If I worked too much, she made me take time off. I could never go very long without a subtle (or not so subtle) reminder to take my medicine. I wondered if my mother had called Linda and asked her to hound me. Mom hadn't called of course—Linda simply cared.

Lori: Setting the Bar High

After my divorce, I wasn't open to dating. I grew comfortable with being single and living without a girlfriend. I wanted to focus on building my career and staying active with hiking, skiing, and mountain biking. My self-confidence was at an all-time low because I had failed to keep the one woman I had loved. Like most trying times of my life, however, a special person just happened to come along at a seemingly perfect time. One of my best clients was a travel agent, who eventually introduced me to a hotel saleswoman named Lori. Although Lori was my business competitor, we were immediately attracted to each other. On the recommendation of my friend, I ended up inviting Lori to attend a huge party my hotel was hosting for the John Elway Foundation. Many top sports celebrities had attended past events, and the celebrity list for this year was no exception. I had management duties that night for a few hours, so I introduced Lori to a few people. This would give her a few "fall back" people to socialize with while I was intermittently called away to take care of guests. I was still concerned she might not have a good time, as she didn't know anybody. Each time I checked in with her, however, she was the center of the conversation; she was always talking to someone new and they seemed to love her. About midway through the evening, I was free from work duties—and it couldn't have been too soon, as *I* wanted to be the guy she was talking with!

I understood immediately why she made such an incredible impression on everyone. She was smart, charming, beautiful, and easy to talk to. We began a dating relationship in which she set new rules of engagement. We didn't have anything real to fight about, so we didn't make things harder for each other by bringing home "junk" from our workdays. Life is going to throw you enough junk without your making up stuff.

When she bought a house in Denver, she needed to furnish it. We hadn't been dating long, so I didn't know what to get her. Too expensive a gift, and I was over-committing. Too little a gift, and I was cheap. I liked her tremendously, so I wanted to get something good. In the end I decided to buy her a ficus tree. She had said she needed a plant or two, and it wasn't the cheapest thing in the world—besides, what did I know about furniture, carpets, and wall fixtures? I felt very awkward at the gift and jokingly expressed that to her. Her words immediately put me at great ease and gave me the confidence to once again be myself. She said: I know who you are. You were raised in a family of boys. You are a man's man and I like that about you. Don't worry, it is a perfect gift. With her simple reassurance, she made me confident again and allowed me to truly be me and begin healing.

It was too soon after my divorce, however, for our relationship to truly take hold. I was not ready to return to that kind of genuine care for another. I was wrapped up in my own world and couldn't give enough in return. There are two things I will be forever grateful to Lori for: she let me know that it was okay to be myself, and more importantly, she set higher expectations of what it would take to find and keep a person of her caliber in my life.

Leslie: My Greatest Humiliation and Lesson

One of my best friends is a runner and a woman. She is also my "arch-enemy," as you will find out later. We met while running and have spent hundreds of hours side by side, keeping each other company while training for races. I have the privilege of being the person who encouraged her to begin competing in endurance races.

For a long time I ran by myself. After meeting Leslie, I learned running with another person could make the miles go by faster and that they would be more enjoyable. Running with someone also creates a bit of competition, even if you are both laid back. When we first started running, I held the fastest time between us. We regularly compared notes for 5 miles, 13.1 miles, and 26.2 miles. I was proud to say I was the faster between us. As Leslie started to run more and more, eventually completing her first marathon, our friendly competition intensified. I thought it right and proper that I should hold the faster times since I was the more experienced runner, but her times were nipping at my heels.

Each year we ran the St. Patricks' Day race, which is five miles long. After a couple years of this, we really wanted to put in a special effort and shatter our fastest times. We trained hard and met up at the starting line. Our pace was blistering for the first 3.5 miles. Soon I was struggling to keep up, and then *couldn't* keep up. Leslie started to pull away and I soon lost sight of her. Approaching the final hill I got a second wind, and before I knew it, I saw Leslie just ahead. With just 100 meters or so to go we were side by side. I had given every ounce of effort to catch her, and I would retain bragging rights between us for the 5-mile distance. Although I didn't beat her, we did finish literally side by side. Afterward, as we were talking about the race, I asked what happened to her toward the end. After all, she had pulled away and then slowed down significantly. Her answer was a blow to my male ego. She said: "I wanted us to finish together, so I slowed down for you!" Well, that was the beginning of the end. Leslie now owns the best times in all race distances.

All ego and joking aside, I am so proud of her and thankful that running brought us together. We have run so many races together, including the 2007 Marine Corp Marathon. Much like the St. Patrick's Day race, I fell behind her early. Late in the race I spotted her just a few runners ahead of me. Unlike St.

Patrick's Day, she did not slow down for me. (Once again, beat by a girl!) I like the nature of our little competition, though; it drives me to press on and put in the hard work to keep up with her. What I get out of our runs together is so much more than exercise.

Leslie married a great guy named Dave and they have two beautiful children. Rene and Leslie became instant friends, as I had hoped for. How lucky I am to have such great women in my life, even if they sometimes crush my ego on race day!

I have most certainly received the most support in life from women; and that's a fact that I didn't realize in my youth. Only in adulthood did I acknowledge the all-important support and love that is uniquely feminine.

Chapter 16

A PARTNER

*"Love is revealing to someone else
that person's own beauty."*

Jean Vanier, Catholic humanitarian

Rene's Story

My wife is an incredible combination of strength, passion, tenderness, and joy. It seems every time I explain her to someone, I always start out with strength. I often describe her toughness first; the strength and toughness I refer to is internal. All of the compassion, love, and tenderness in the world wouldn't hold up our relationship without the power that lies beneath it all. In joining her life to mine, she committed to a life that was not going to be the easiest. How does such a beautiful and strong woman come to be? Let me tell you...

Rene was born and raised in small towns across the Midwest and South. She was born in Champaign, Illinois, and lived there for a few years with her mother, Donna. She never had the opportunity to know her father, because shortly after her birth he left to pursue a career in racecar driving. Unable or unwilling to face the demands of fatherhood, he would not be a part of her life again. Rene's mother wanted to be near her family, so she moved to Russell Springs, Kentucky. Much of Rene's early years were spent in Russell Springs, where she spent a wonderful childhood. Many relatives from her mom's side of the family, including her grandma, were there to be a part of her life. Being an outgoing and energetic girl, Rene made many friends.

Donna eventually remarried; Rene's stepfather was a military man. He was a captain in the Army Reserves and attached to Fort Campbell. He decided to move to active duty and was transferred to Louisiana. After a few years in Louisiana, his final transfer was to St. Louis, MO. This final move happened just as Rene started high school—and that's where our stories begin to converge. Rene attended St. Charles West High School. St. Charles was not a big city (it has since expanded quite a bit), so most kids grew up together and at some point at least played on the same sports teams. All the neighborhood kids I grew up with went to St. Charles West. Rene and I don't remember ever meeting, however. That's odd, since we knew all of the same people. She even dated one of my neighbors.

Rene wanted to get out of town right after high school. Although she did well in school and had ambitions of attending college, her stepfather had no intention of helping her out financially. Rather, he encouraged her to consider entering the military. Rene did like what she had heard during a military interview, and she decided to enter the Air Force.

After basic training, Rene was off to England for four years. Upon returning to the U.S. after four years in the Air Force, Rene was very anxious to improve herself by going to college. The G.I. bill was useful, but it only paid for so much. If nothing else, Rene is practical, so she started classes at the local community college. Earning top academic honors became a habit for her. Rene ended up finishing her four-year college degree at a highly respected university, once again earning top academic honors. She did this while working full-time for two years, then working full-time as an intern. Naturally, the internship was at one of St. Louis's top companies. Her systematic and detailed approach to all things in life were lining up perfectly for her eventual career in software quality assurance, and later in project management. She is a perfect compliment to my off-the-cuff and "adventurous" approach to all things.

Upon moving back to St. Louis, both Rene and I reconnected with old friends. We had a lot of fun memories from our youth, and renewing those friendships was familiar and exciting. In the midst of spending more time with these mutual friends, we were finally introduced. One night I was invited to a birthday party and it just happened that Rene was going to be with "the crowd." I had either grown up, gone to high school, or gone to college with the crowd, so Rene and I were introduced as if we should automatically know one another. We didn't recognize each other, though, so we just became casual acquaintances.

It wasn't easy getting to know each other during that time. Rene had just finished college and was very focused on building her career and gaining independence. There was another small detail—she had a boyfriend. With her busy life and my world already being centered on training for marathons, we remained very casual acquaintances. The typical outing with "the gang" consisted of everyone going out to dinner followed by extending the night out with cocktails, dancing, and such. There were also occasional concerts and parties that everyone went to. That would leave plenty of time for us to find each other—but my typical outing with the gang was different. I would typically go to dinner and then go straight home. I needed to relax a bit and go to bed early. I liked to hang out with the gang, sure, but my training took precedence over everything. I must have seemed boring, crazy, and obsessed (or maybe all three!).

Finally Together

After a couple years of this, I finally had the chance to stay out late. In October of 2002, I was invited to Rene's brother-in-law's birthday party. I was excited to go out, because for the first time in two years I wasn't training for a marathon when everyone was going out on the town. As a matter of fact, I had just run the Chicago Marathon the weekend before. I had had a really good race and was ready to celebrate. Nearly twenty of us sat down for dinner, and Rene noticed that she and I were the only single people. (She had recently broken up with her boyfriend.) She laughingly said she didn't want to be sitting by herself with all the other couples, but I really knew she wanted to sit next to me. (At least, that is what I kept telling myself!) We sat next to each other at dinner and we began to talk in-depth. As I suspected, we knew many of the same people. We could even recall specific parties in high school we were both at. I knew most of her friends well, but for the life of me, I couldn't pinpoint her in my past. It was perplexing but fun to start putting our commonalities together. I was starting to like her.

When the Girl is Right, the Time Will Be Right

As the night went on, I didn't want to leave her. The more I learned about her, the more I wanted to know. I remember three things from that night that impressed me most: she had lived overseas and served our country while I was going to keg parties. She put herself through college when I had help from mom and dad. Finally, she owned a Corvette and was a huge sports nut. That was a combination of life experience and personality I had not met in anyone else before. I had to get to know her more. I was trying to decide about the appropriate time to call to ask her out. The next day? Three days? One week? I would play the "dating game" and try to be cool. In the end, though, I'm so not cool and besides, I didn't want to play games. I called her the next day and asked if she would like to go to dinner. I was so excited when she said yes. I can't remember a day, in the 11 years since, when we have not spoken to each other.

I liked her tremendously within just a few short months. I wasn't completely sure where our relationship was going; as a matter of fact, I had a dilemma. It was now early January, and in March the gang was going to Colorado together for a ski trip. My dilemma was this: if we're dating, but it isn't serious, it might be awkward to be on a trip together for a week. If we break up, we will be stuck in the same car and same house for a week together, and that will *definitely* be awkward!

By late January, however, I had no intention of letting her go anywhere without me. In a few short months my admiration for her grew tremendously. I learned about her military career. I liked that she was not afraid to be away from her home. While based overseas, she had made it a point to travel throughout Europe. I really loved that because I also highly enjoy adventure. After the military years, she lived with her younger sister and mother while putting herself through college. I was also close to my own family. Finally, she was a devoted sports fan. Baseball was her favorite, but she enjoyed sports of all kinds. What impressed me most was how independent yet how loving she was.

Breaking The Shell

Having been divorced as well, Rene struggled with how she would fit into someone's life again. She also didn't have much to be positive about when it came to men in general. Her ex-husband had violated her trust in a most hurtful way and her biological father had bowed out of her life. She had every reason in the world to be overly cautious. I could sense the distrust within her, and from time to time she would express it in an indirect way. It worried me because I so wanted to be a part of her life. In my opinion, she had earned the right to have the very best man in her life. Even though there was a barrier created by these experiences, she was incredibly warm and loyal and I was hoping to live up to the high expectations she must have had.

I wanted to get past her "edge." When she said she didn't need a man to define her, I knew that to be true and was relieved to know she had that strength in her; but I also wanted her to know that I was ready for her and was hoping she was ready for me. On a trip to see her family in Illinois, I asked if we could talk more about her statement about men. I told her that I knew she didn't need a man to take care of her. I told her I didn't want to be taken care of. Nor did I feel the need to take care of her. However, what I did desire was someone who *wanted* to be with me. I wanted someone who would be my partner in life, so we could support one another.

On a side note, I find it interesting that the word *partner* has a relatively unknown definition. **Part • ner**: *One of the heavy timbers that strengthens a ship's deck to support a mast.* Just to be clear, I don't consider myself and Rene to be pieces of timber. This obscure definition of *partner* tells you what Rene is to my life. I needed someone strong enough, mentally and

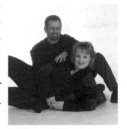

Mike and Rene

spiritually, to handle life with a chronic illness. Someone with the strength to be independent when it was called for and someone who wouldn't let me slack when I wanted to. Someone who could handle a not-so-ordinary life. I wanted someone with that unique blend of strength, independence, loyalty, and love. Without a partner, the ship doesn't sail. My desire to have a partner rang true with Rene. From that point forward, we moved together as a team.

United by Running

If you ever watch the old TV sitcom *Friends,* you may recall the episode when Rachel and Phoebe are running together. Rachel is running normally, looking like a pro. Phoebe, however, is running wildly with arms flailing and legs flying out to the side. Are you picturing a little kid running uncontrollably down a hill? That is what Rene looked like the first time we ran together. (Ok, I exaggerate, but not by much.) It was the spring of 2004 and we were running together for the very first time. The previous year, in June, Rene went to her first marathon as a spectator. That was my third marathon and the first one with Rene in my life.

Planning for marathons is fun. Your first priority is looking to see which races have a good reputation for being fast and well-organized. The second consideration is the weather. The third factor for a serious runner is: what city are we visiting? Going to Chicago, New York, or another cool city is a real bonus, but not the ultimate prize. For the *spectator,* the three priorities are reversed. I had told Rene that my choice was either Grandma's Marathon in Duluth, Minnesota, or the San Diego Marathon. For a spectator, the choice was easy! Who wouldn't want to soak up the sun and go to the ocean? When I told her we were actually going to the Midwest, icebox town of Duluth, she was in disbelief. Both marathons had good reputations, but I had heard much more about Grandma's. It always ranked in the top ten most favorite marathons in anything I read. Being ever supportive, though, Rene went along with my enthusiasm.

We had a wonderful trip to Duluth. The town was actually very interesting. The people of Duluth treated the marathoners like royalty. The night before the race we went to have dinner, and downtown Duluth was packed with runners. On race day, Rene was situated near the finish line. She got caught up in the spirit of what running 26.2 miles was like. Later, the night of race day, I was recovering and in typical fashion barely able to move. The combination of seeing my preparation first-hand, watching thousands of runners struggling the last few steps, and observing the physical toll it took on me gave Rene a fresh perspective on the sport. From that day on, she was completely supportive of my running endeavors and became my main "cheerleader."

Rene was genuinely intrigued by the marathon experience. She was also curious about the social aspect of running. I was constantly talking about the cool people I was always getting to know. In the summer of 2004, Rene's curiosity and goal-driven personality took over. She wanted to do a half marathon! So, we began by going for a little jog. While I was watching my form for efficiency, Rene was running like it was a 100-meter sprint—with no form. Within a quarter mile, she was spent. Totally out of breath, she was frustrated and a bit embarrassed.

Now, I've been told you don't want to teach your spouse anything. I've been told it could ruin your relationship, so a husband or wife should just leave things alone or hire professional help. I couldn't help myself, so I asked if I could give her a few pointers on how to run. She was wondering: what is there to learn about running? One foot in front of the other, right? Well, I thought, there is quite a lot to know when you want to run 13.1 miles without stopping. Being the awesome person she is, Rene listened to me with an open mind. She quickly started increasing her mileage, but she still didn't feel like she was a runner because she was "slow" and didn't look like an Olympic marathoner. I continued to encourage her, however, because I knew from personal experience that just as Rome wasn't built in a day, no marathon runner is made overnight.

That September, I was running a half marathon in our hometown. Rene volunteered at a water station at the race and got to see me run by. She also observed the many other runners completing the race. Previously, all runners in her mind had looked like my marathon friends and me: skinny! No matter what I told her about her own ability to run, she saw it as impossible. That day, she saw lots of runners, and they sure weren't all beanpole skinny. As a matter of fact, the runners completing that half marathon were all sorts of people that didn't look like a typical runner. Being involved in that race and seeing everything first-hand gave Rene a new confidence that she too could complete her goal.

With the goal of a half marathon in her sights, it was Rene's turn to pick a city. You could pretty much guarantee that we were going someplace "cool." Within six months of our first awkward and tiring jog, we went to Disney World and ran the 2005 Disney Half Marathon. Disney World in January is a nice little getaway. Plus, she did awesome! With her mom and sister at the finishing line, it was a perfect day.

By this time, I was head-over-heels in love with this woman and wanted to propose to her. I visited her mother and expressed how much Rene meant to me. With her mother's backing, I hatched a scheme to propose. I thought it would be an excellent surprise to be at the finish line with her ring and propose right there at Disney World. Upon further consideration, I thought that might not be as romantic as imagined. What if she hated the half-marathon experience? Her memories of our engagement would not be fond. In reality, I knew she would be tired, sweaty and sore at that point, so I thought: let's take one good thing at a time. A few weeks before the race, on Christmas morning, I hung an engagement ring from a ribbon on the Christmas tree. I told her I had bought her an extra present and that it was on the tree. Rene loves ornaments, and I let her think it was a new ornament. When she couldn't find the new ornament amongst all the shiny decorations, I had to guide her to the surprise. When she saw it and cried tears of joy, I had my answer!

Not being one to stop at one race, Rene set a goal of completing another half marathon. By the fall of 2005, she had finished the Lewis and Clark Half Marathon in St. Charles and had reduced her time by 16:00 minutes. Now she officially had running fever—she set her mind on the 2006 Chicago Marathon. This was no 13.1-mile jog; this was the full 26.2. With her usual tenacity, Rene set forth on a new fitness goal. By the end of 2007 she was coaching with Fleet Feet Sports and had completed six or so half marathons and two full marathons. (Do I love this woman, or what?)

While we were not running side-by-side, we did have something else in common. Four or so days a week, we would drive over to a park for our run. Running gave us a lot to talk about. It was important to me that all my "running friends" were now her friends. The friends she was gaining by running became *my* friends. After a few years of coaching, we had some of the best people to call friends. Running isn't really Rene's "thing," but she is goal-driven and is quite sociable, so having a community of driven yet highly personable runners was working out well. Accomplishing a goal like finishing 26.2 miles is also confidence boosting, and she was brimming with confidence after her Chicago run. We were having fun! I believe running also gave her new perspective on how difficult it was for me to be running marathons. She knows first hand the drive, dedication, and perseverance that are required to run endurance races.

At the same time, I know it is a bit difficult to be married to me. Aside from the challenge of just putting up with me, she has to endure the strong drive I have to be adventurous and push my abilities to the limit. Attempting marathons and triathlons requires hours and hours of training time each week. That means I am swimming, biking, and running quite a bit. All that time is cutting into our personal time together. Doing all these things is not inexpensive, either. She also understands, however, that it's not just about staying healthy. She knows a huge part of that exercise is about me knowing I'm fighting this disease on *my* terms. She knows that it's a positive way for me to "embrace" my life with a chronic illness.

Many runners have told us that their spouse is not supportive of their running. They tell us it's a battle to escape the house for a few hours because their spouse is griping. This is not something we understand from personal experience. I always tell these friends to let their spouses know how important it is; I encourage my friends to tell their spouses that running is quite mind clearing. Running obviously makes the body stronger. (It also makes the body sexier, and who can complain about that?) My favorite response for the unhappy spouse of a runner is telling them that without running to blow off steam, she/he wouldn't be able to tolerate you! (Only half-jokingly, of course.) I suppose it all boils down to perspective. Rene and I have the benefit of looking at exercise as a life-or-death deal. We don't have to look years down the road; our reality is more acute. If I don't exercise, we can hear it in my lungs in a very short time. We can't change that perspective, so we've learned how to benefit from it.

Rene has been my partner for 11 years. I have more peace than I'd imagined possible. She is the rock upon which our little family is built. I've learned to step back and simply watch her go. When I'm bummed out, she's there. When I'm overjoyed, she's there. When I'm scheming the next adventure, she is there. I am amazed at how loving and purpose-driven she remains, especially given the early fatherly role models she endured. Rene drives me to be better. She inspires me to push myself. She comforts the unease that lies beneath.

Absolute Love

To remain in love can be a real challenge. Life is constantly tugging at our bonds. Work, money, and health seem to destroy the bonds of marriage with too much frequency. To this point, our struggles have made us stronger. I have more respect and admiration for Rene now than I did 11 years ago. In a weird way, we are constantly reminded of why we love one another. Blessings, disguised in a chronic illness, have helped us to not take each other for granted. We have been interviewed for many news articles, TV news stories, documentaries, and fund raising videos. Each time, I get to tell the story of how I fell in love with Rene and what she means to me every day. Fortunately for me, Rene also gets to tell the cameras why she loves me so much. We need constant reminders of these things, because life tends to get in the way of our bonds. Maybe every married couple should hire a filmmaker or journalist to visit their house and ask why they fell in love. They could ask what it feels like when their spouse does the small things or comes through in a difficult moment. Maybe that should happen on an annual basis so we can clear the fog from our minds and hearts and see our love for one another more clearly.

Chapter 17

ELEVEN LONG YEARS

"Patience, young grasshopper."

Kung Fu, TV show [1972-1975]

For eleven years, from 2001 to 2012, I got to experience spectacular feelings of conquering my life's challenges. For the most part, I had gained control of my life, or at least the attitude I approached life with. I chose a job that didn't overwhelm my time and eventually started my own business, which gave me ultimate control over my time. I was nearly 100% *compliant* with the various medicines and therapies that had to be taken. I made a conscious effort to eat better and live a more fulfilled life through tackling my battle head-on.

Since there are not many people my age with this disease, we are a small group and really don't know what to expect. We are essentially lab rats when it comes to living through middle age. Since there are even fewer exercising with the vigorous regimen I maintain, the "unknown" is even greater in my case. The goal of doctors treating my condition is to slow down the decline of lung function and keep it to the "predicted" rate that the general population experiences. What is "normal" lung capacity for my condition at my age is unknown, so I really didn't know if exercise was paying off—other than the mental benefits, which were certain. I was hoping that all the exercise would at least keep my lung functions steady, but little by little they were declining.

Still, I was confident because I was actively fighting off the worst possibilities of this disease and actually having fun doing it. On the other hand, I was frustrated because I was still losing vital lung capacity. It was difficult for me to see other people gaining back once-lost lung capacity. It wasn't difficult because I was jealous; it was quite the opposite. As I read stories from around the country of this person or that who had a great success story of healing their lungs, I was hopeful it would someday happen for me. Eleven years of running, running, and more running. Eleven years of getting to every doctor appointment and staying highly compliant. Not perfectly compliant, but very nearly so. I knew I was doing good things for my body and mind by exercising vigorously, but there was no reward of increased lung function.

In the tenth year of this regimen, I was at the lowest level of lung capacity ever: 63% of a normal 42-year-old. Sixty-three percent of normal. Reverse that: 37% of my lungs' ability to process oxygen was gone. In the summer of 2011, I could very much feel this decreased capacity. I was out of breath at running paces that should have been easy; I tired much more quickly on the bike. I could feel shortness of breath at exercise levels that should have been routine. I didn't question *why* I was still exercising so much, because it was tremendous mental therapy just to be doing something active. I was frustrated, however, that my lung levels continued to drop just a little bit each time I went the doctor.

Over that past decade or so, I had to continually set a goal. If I was not registered for a race, my exercise work was harder to finish. I felt like a slacker at times, but soon found out that most of us are wired this way. Many runners and triathletes I speak with stay motivated by having the next race (or two) lined up. Now, these people are certainly not slackers. Most people who plan to tackle a 3-hour marathon or an Ironman Triathlon are not slackers. I felt I was in good company, even when I felt motivation ebbing. In order to stay motivated, I kept signing up for the next race. The worse I did in a race, the more quickly I signed up for the next one.

Over the span of time I was competing in these races, I felt the limitations of my body many times over. I fell down. I had to walk. I even had a DNF (Did Not Finish), which was emotionally painful, because the many months of training culminated in what felt like an epic failure. To add to my emotional turmoil, when that DNF happened I had already registered for a 60-mile bike race, which was to take place not long after that.

Why re-enlist after a crushing failure? Because I was not going to accept that that was how things would be. Not enrolling in the next race would mean admitting that my spirit was crushed. In each race, whether it ended in a personal record or a DNF, I was testing my will. While I found the limitations of my body, I have yet to find the limitations of my will. I hope I never do.

You may find this a dangerous game, to push one's willpower to the max. What happens if I find my limit, you may ask? My question in return is: why operate out of fear of "what if?" I did that for long enough, and the "what if" never happened. Why not operate with the notion that testing your will is like testing your body? You work out your body to make it stronger. Let me make an analogy to weight lifting: you can't lift heavier weights without lifting heavier weights. In order to increase the weight one can lift, you have to "max out." Essentially, we are finding the maximum tolerance of our muscles in order to push through to the next level. Running is the same—as is any challenge in life. Even academics is the same: you can't jump from simple addition and subtraction to calculus. There is (sometimes painful) stretching of your knowledge in the form of multiplication tables and long division and progression to algebra and geometry and beyond. Everything is like this. If we never push a bit, we will never stretch a bit.

What I found is that when I received bad news, my willpower was ready. I was diagnosed with ulcers, and we approached it as just one more thing to take care of. I was diagnosed with diabetes—just one more thing to manage. I was hospitalized, once resulting in a nearly 20% drop in lung function in 5 days. Just one more thing to work hard to overcome. For 11 years I saw an incremental drop in lung functions, yet I persisted in staying the course.

I didn't just have stubborn willpower and "make it through" attitude. I was absolutely bent on embracing each new challenge and doing my best with what my body was giving. Was I frustrated each time I got bad news? You bet. Did I get angry? Yes! Did I get sad? Did I use some "choice words" in an internal dialogue? Always! Did I quit? *Never!* (Did I make sure I was registered for another race to give me focus? ABSOLUTELY!)

Here's the kicker: there are times when I'm struggling to stay motivated and positive. If I didn't have something to focus on, I would quit and probably turn bitter. Find your *something*. Find your reason to get out of bed and take the medicine, and live for that reason. Is it sports of some kind? Is it business? Is it family? Is it serving others? Is it academics? Is it a deeper spiritual life? Is it chess or checkers? The "it" doesn't matter. What matters is finding the thing that gets you fired up and encourages you to stretch beyond what you ever expected. Don't forget: none of the above matters if you're dead—so don't forget that you have to manage your health. In addition to the practice of "stretching your abilities," you should also put in action internal "affirming words." Thinking positive thoughts and speaking positive words are an excellent starting point for embracing your challenge. It can't stop there, however, because words and thoughts are fine, but the world doesn't change without *action*. In order for you to do well in life, you have to dig deep and find the willpower to make it through tough circumstances. Without digging deep into your will and truly changing yourself with action, positive talk and affirmations are empty promises to yourself.

Three years ago, my lung capacity was at 63%. That is a lousy number, and I was worried and frustrated. I kept working at it, though, not always having 100% confidence I would stop the slide, much less rebound. At this lowest point in my health, I readjusted expectations. Maybe marathons and Ironmans were out of the picture for me. Maybe I would have to just run 10k races or sprint triathlons. I might even have to do them slowly. I became comfortable with the notion that I would still run, bike, and swim, although be it at a slower pace. (Heck, we all get older and slow down anyway!) There was no way I was quitting, though. I relied on the willpower that was built during those 11 years, and stayed with my exercise goals.

Payload

There is a happy ending to that chapter of my life—since October of 2011, my lung capacity has actually been on the increase. Testing my lungs over the past couple years, my doctor has confirmed my lung capacity as high as 97%. That is nearly normal. The disease I have is progressive, and we not only halted the progression, but reversed it. We tried new drugs and I stayed 100% compliant and kept with the exercise plans. Eleven years of strengthening my body and mind had finally paid off!

I'm glad I pushed and stretched. Through those 11 years, so many great things happened. I met new people that gave me encouragement. I was presented with the opportunity to give encouragement many times, and maybe even help change the course of someone's life. I experienced many times over what it felt like to be victorious and overcome odds. I gained a deeper understanding of myself and became more compassionate toward others. That's not what I set off to do with my long-ago decision to move home to St. Louis and regain my physical health; my goal was simply to become happier and healthier. Who knew there was so much more in store for me? I certainly didn't see it then.

Keep this in mind: if your "A" plan for life doesn't seem to be working out… don't worry. It may just mean you are destined for greater things that you can't envision just now. Plan B is even better!

Chapter 18

BEYOND ME

*"Consider it all joy, my brethren,
when you encounter various trials,
knowing that the testing of your faith
produces endurance. And let
endurance have its perfect result,
so that you may be perfect and
complete, lacking in nothing."*

James, an early Christian

It has been a number of years since my fateful 30th birthday and the decision to make a real difference in my life. I knew something special was happening, because I had more peace of mind than ever before. I had moved from purely "survival mode" to "thriving mode," which freed my mind to explore who I truly was. As a kid, and through my twenties and early thirties, I had plenty of people try to tell something to the effect of the above Bible quote. I heard that my challenges would bring me closer to God. When I heard something like that, I would immediately discount anything else that person had to say. I considered them to be some version of crazy, or at best, I was suspicious of them as just another "Bible-thumping" person out of touch with reality. However, later in life, I came to be more open to hearing spiritual advice from others. While these first few sentences of the book of James speak directly about one's spiritual life, I have come to realize it also applies to the fight to stay healthy and motivated.

Through running, I found a great way to begin to overcome my challenges in life. By the time I was 32, I was enjoying physical health by any standard. Mentally and emotionally, I had also done a 180-degree turnaround and no longer made decisions based on negative thoughts or fear. As a matter of fact, I had wrapped my arms around life and begun to embrace every aspect of it. Using the tool of running to tackle personal demons was proving a wonderful thing. During one long run of double-digit miles it dawned on me, however, that I might not always be able to run or even walk. These thoughts were not negative or fearful in nature; they were more of an internal reflection. My question was: where would I be if my health deteriorated and I could no longer do the thing that had helped me so much? Thinking about that left me back at square one: being frustrated, feeling alone, and getting by without purpose. Through my constant dedication to a better life and overcoming these obstacles, I was beginning to get to know myself. Still, I felt I was only scratching the surface of who I was. I also was very proud of myself for taking the "bull by the horns" and working diligently to overcome my fears. I had persevered. I had motivated myself. I was succeeding on my own terms.

More internal searching was taking place, however, and I had to admit I was only a part of this newfound attitude and life view. The more I thought about things, the more I was willing to admit that there were a great deal of people surrounding me from the moment I was born to the present day who filled my life with something very special. My internal dialogue turned more and more away from *me* and opened up to the possibilities of something bigger. I let my thoughts simmer. The more I read and listened, the more I realized that the best advice about living with great challenges had already been written a long, long time ago. The quote at the beginning of this chapter, and many other passages from the Bible, started to make much more sense to me. In particular, I was attracted to the theme of difficult circumstances leading to a greater good. It is something we hear and want to believe, but when "difficult" is playing out in our lives, this concept is not usually welcome and often not comforting.

I had already experienced this first hand, though, and what hit me square between the eyes was this realization: the very *hardest* activity for me to do to ensure good health was the very *best* thing I could do for my health. My compromised body, that actually has no business running, benefits the most from this particular activity. I continued to listen to my internal dialogue and to open up to possibilities. I couldn't help but ask: how could such a simple people as those in the first century have known what we know now in the 21st century? Even living without all the scientific and intellectual advancements of our age, did these people of ancient times still have valuable life lessons to teach me?

There were still many unanswered questions about my future. While the anxiety and decision-making based on a negative future were gone, there was still a hollow place inside me. The hole consisted of these questions: what kind of life is this, having to deal with the daily grind of a chronic illness? Why do I have to deal with this while others have a "perfect" life? Is this just a grind, just getting by, without any greater purpose? During one time of organized spiritual reflection, I was asked to say any prayer that came to mind. I thought a lot about this question. What would I pray for? Would I ask for something? Would I simply give praise to God? Would I petition for the well being of a loved one? In the end, what came pouring out was simply gratitude. I was thankful for my wife, my parents, my brothers, and my friends. I was thankful for an adventurous spirit. I was thankful for the fortitude, perseverance, and positive attitude I was humbled to have been given. (Let's not forget: I also must always be thankful for devilishly handsome good looks.) Joking aside, these were the answers uppermost in my mind, but I still felt they were not precisely hitting the target. What else was I thankful for?

When it got right down to it, I was thankful for the very thing that made all the great things in my life possible: life itself. For the first time in 34 years, I honestly said that I was thankful for my life. The life full of thousands of pills, coughing, stomachaches, anxious moments and challenges was a real blessing and not the curse I felt it was for so many years. I find it ironic that the very thing I rejected for so many years was right in front of my face as my greatest blessing, and summed up in a couple of sentences by James, a man who had lived in a time very different from mine. I had endured. I endured many trials: physical, emotional, and spiritual. I was tested on many levels, and by finding joy in life instead of being bitter and angry, I had "lacked nothing" to that point.

I continue to pray that my life remains full of good things. In particular, I pray that if things turn in a different direction, I remain joyful even in the face of new challenges. My last thought regarding James is that although I sometimes think I am perfect, I must admit I'm not. Perfection is a noteworthy goal, though, and I will always strive for it: "Be ye therefore perfect, even as your heavenly Father is perfect." (Matthew 5:48) Since that day of running when I began to ask those questions, and as a result of the continuous reflection I have undergone, I have come to realize the greatest things in life:

1. *My life has a great purpose that reaches beyond the daily grind of taking care of myself.*
2. *The challenges I experience build the best parts of me.*
3. *The challenges I experience build the best things in those around me.*
4. *If my "A Plan" doesn't work out, there is something greater in store for me that I just might not be able to see yet.*
5. *The best advice written on how to live a life more connected to my fellow humans and stay connected to the purpose beyond myself has already been written, and it was written by average people like James. (Of course, working with some big-time inspiration.) These people knew what hard times were, and God let them in on some big ideas.*

No circumstance or person has ultimate control over you; *you* are the one calling the shots in your life. The more I get in touch with the teachings of Jesus Christ, the more my life makes sense and has more purpose than I could discover on my own or through others. What I can tell you is that I work every day to live with greater purpose and appreciation for ALL things in my life. For me, the biggest turn-around was moving away from selfish thoughts of what *I* thought I was missing to outwardly directed thoughts on what I could give back to my fellow human beings. I thought not being able to father children was a sad fact of living with my disease. Now I know I can adopt, foster, or volunteer for children who need a supportive male figure in their lives. I thought this burden of a chronic disease had no purpose. Now I know that this disease puts me in a very unique position to understand others who need encouragement.

At first, I allowed this sickness to separate me from God. I now see that Jesus opened the way to life with Him in a very specific way, by giving up His life for me, and in a bloody, humiliating, and painful way. That ultimate act of humility shows us that life, even with challenges, can be filled with dignity and tremendous purpose. I can't bring the level of Christ's redemption to the world, but maybe just a sliver of that redemption is in store for all of us who live with great challenges. I thought I would be alone in my struggles, but Jesus constantly calls us to come to the side of others. Because I have this disease, I see a constant parade of charity and compassion, and I am humbled by the presence of God manifesting itself through the people around me.

Whether you believe Jesus Christ is the Son of God or you believe he was simply a philosopher who lived a long time ago, His teachings are packed full of wisdom on how to live with great purpose. His teachings always encourage us to embrace our challenges and the challenges of others. He outlines an inspiring way to live and undeniably one to strive for.

I find the depths of the teaching in the Bible matches the depth of the search for something greater in life. Sometimes the wisdom of Biblical verses seems simplistic at first. But when I reflect on them, they become complex and deep. When I try to live them out, I have yet more challenges to overcome; but I see the fruit in the effort both for myself and for those I come in contact with. This challenge of living an upright life sometimes feels harder than managing my disease, but because it's difficult, I know it will bear good fruit.

Chapter 19

MY CHALLENGE

"The greater the obstacle, the more glory in overcoming it."

Molière, French playwright and actor

If you're like all my past girlfriends and the occasional curious caveman, you may have already researched the symptoms I have been telling you about. By now you may know what my disease is—I was born with cystic fibrosis (CF).

Like many serious illnesses, the effects of CF are not always visible. In my own case, I often have to convince others I actually have a seriously messed-up body. I have to impress upon them the vast amounts of medicine I take and that my exercise, at its core, is therapy. To the untrained eye, the physical effects of my disease are not obvious. One might notice our underweight figures, as most people with my condition struggle to maintain a healthy weight. "Clubbed fingernails," which are misshapen and obvious to us, are rarely noticed by others. Only when the disease's progression is severe enough do you take notice. Then, you can't miss it: that very distinct-sounding cough of a person with CF. The cough that comes from deep within the lungs as the body desperately tries to work an infected substance out. My doctor has said that the speed at which air is moved through the lungs when coughing approaches the speed of sound. That is pretty amazing. (It's amazing that we don't blow ourselves right off our feet!) It is also horrifying that even at that speed and force, my body still cannot get the "junk" out of my lungs without serious medicine and therapy.

With an untrained eye and ear, you would never guess that there is a problem, unless you're lucky enough to be in earshot of someone with CF coughing. Because CF and some other conditions are "hidden," sometimes people around us have a hard time relating to the difficulties of the person dealing with our condition. We end up putting people on an island. There it is again—the island. It's one thing to put yourself there, but another thing to put someone else there by your actions.

There was a controversy some months ago about a child who was forced to miss a school function because he had too many absences. The school withheld the boy (who suffered from CF) from some fun activities at school because he had missed many days due to his poor health. The mother of this child brought the issue to the attention of the local news, and a lot of conversation—not all of it supportive—was held. The more I think about it, the sometimes-dismissive reaction of the public also applies to other misunderstood or unseen medical conditions.

Social media went crazy talking about the news story, and one person said that the boy "needs to toughen up" because "life isn't fair" and kids "aren't learning life lessons any longer." To this person I wanted to say: no kidding, life isn't fair, but who are we to "toughen up" a kid who's going to get a lifetime of "unfair" up to his eyeballs. I really don't know if this mom was "right" or the school was "right." I was just surprised that the vast majority of comments were in the vein that the kid was going to have to suck it up. Man, that is brutal, I thought. Life is really quite hard enough already, without unknowing people making it even more difficult. What is really ironic for all the people who commented so ignorantly is this: that kid will undoubtedly become the toughest kid on the block. If he survives to adulthood, he will be stronger than all the knuckleheads trying to "teach him a lesson."

I could say all day long that "it's not fair." I must train just as hard as anyone else for marathons, and I get lesser results. Maybe that could be seen as unfair. Really, to me, it just is what it is and I don't desire to make exceptions for myself. The person who feels sorry for me is missing the point. All I ask is: just don't make my life harder than it has to be by being ignorant or dismissive about the difficulties I persist through.

When I was coaching for a half marathon program one summer, one of my runners asked if I got frustrated that this disease makes me a slower runner. She asked if I ever wonder what the possibilities would be if I didn't have cystic fibrosis. My reaction was no, I don't obsess but yes, I wonder. Of course, I would like to run just one mile without coughing. Of course, I would like to go without gas or diarrhea or shortness of breath. I think answering *absolutely no* to her question would be kidding myself. What I told her is that I don't think about it because it's my reality. I asked her to think about how cool it was that I was still in the "1% Club" even if I'm a middle-of-the-pack marathoner. I also asked her to think how cool it was that I wasn't just participating, but I was coaching others and helping them achieve huge personal goals. Finally, I responded by saying that without CF, I would be just another runner in the pack—and isn't it motivating to see other people doing stuff that you take for granted? I'm glad she asked, because I realized I had truly turned my thinking around and maybe even caught a glimpse of my purpose in life.

he•ro•ic
Definition: *Behavior that is bold; brave; of great intensity; very large.*

These are the definitions of *heroic*, and I am surrounded by heroic people. It is bold to embrace the responsibility to raise a child with an uncommon path ahead. It is courageous to protect the smallest among you and to not let anyone mess with him. Being brave is to listen to someone struggling to come to grips with his life when you are just a kid yourself. The many runners striving to achieve a personal goal, with no other prize than a goal achieved, have wills of great intensity. I have seen a great many people with very large hearts get in the fight with me and stand at my side.

I don't have to look far for the great things in life. While your circle of people may look different from mine, I'll bet you don't have to look far either.

For love: I don't have to look past my wife.

For loyalty: My parents, brothers, and in-laws stand close by.

For strength: I see the spouses, friends, and especially loved ones of those we've lost come out in droves to support my fellow CF community.

For grit: I only need to look at my fellow "CFers" doing battle.

For compassion: I show up at a CF fundraiser and see people of all means getting in the fight and giving their resources, time, and energy to a cause.

For commitment and passion: All I have to do is show up at a Saturday morning run. I am surrounded by a bunch of "crazy" marathoners who compete solely for the sake of pushing their abilities. No trophies, no money, no fame; just passion for life and commitment to a goal.

For companionship: My friends are always close at hand and always ready to pitch in.

For financial advice and support: My business colleagues "get" my purpose for being in business and participate in my mission.

The people in my life may have not won an Olympic marathon. They may not have climbed Mt. Everest. They may not have made millions of dollars or been celebrities. These things do not make heroes. What I do know for sure is that the people in my life are the *real deal.*

In this book, I've said a lot and shared many personal stories. My intention is for you, the reader, to realize how much value you bring to the world. No matter what the expectations of your situation are, those circumstances don't have to gain mastery over you. When I hit the rough patches, I remember these things:

- Stay positive. Your positive attitude will draw others to you.
- Challenge attracts; negativity repels. Bitterness chases people away, but hope and strength attract people and their desire to get in the fight with you.
- Internal strength is a must, but the "fortress of solitude" is only for Superman. We must surround ourselves with a loving support network.
- Take action: Action is everything and completes the circle. Thoughts turn into intentions and intentions turn into action, and action produces change.

- Focus on something constructive. Having focus is not running away from your problem. "Focus with purpose" is dealing with your challenge head-on through a constructive outlet. Choose your focus: sports, academics, music, hunting, riding horses. The list could go on forever. Find what excites you, get engaged with it, immerse yourself in it, and surround yourself with people who want to excel at it.
- Be an example: Coach, teach, be an ambassador, or volunteer.
- Join the fight: Find what you have to offer, and offer it. You don't have to be Mother Teresa to make a tremendous impact on someone's world.
- Don't delay: Make a difference now. I've never heard of someone doing something with passion who said they wish they would have waited.

Be heroic! We are made for heroism and cannot be truly happy with anything less.

Thanks for reading my story. I pray for the very best for you.

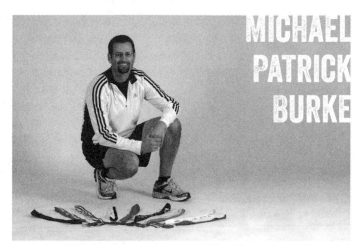

A St. Charles, Missouri native, Mike Burke was diagnosed with a genetic disease at 14 months old—with the expectation that there would likely be no survival beyond childhood.

Mike has changed his mind many times in life. There was only one instance, though, when changing his mind would transform his life. Upon realizing he had wasted many years worrying about his ever-changing but limited life expectancy, Mike decided to never let negative thoughts about living with an incurable and unpredictable disease dictate his life. Growing up with a genetic disease that drastically shortened his life expectancy had blinded him to the possibilities in life. When Mike finally realized that life was full of potential—whether he lived two years or 80 years—his life took on new purpose.

Running 9 full marathons, over 12 half marathons, and competing in a 70.3 Ironman Triathlon is a difficult goal to achieve. There are months of preparation needed. Endurance training takes discipline, perseverance, and patience. For Mike, competing in endurance events with limited lung capacity and having to take over 10,000 pills a year to digest food while managing the onset of a second chronic disease were yet more challenges that he rose to.

WWW.MICHAELPATRICKBURKE.COM